# KETO DIET COOKBOOK

## FOR WOMEN OVER 50

A Simple Guide to a Healthy Lifestyle After Fifty.

Tasty and Easy Low-Carb Ketogenic Recipes to Lose Weight, Detox Your Body, and Balance Hormones

**ELENORE JASLOW**

# TABLE OF CONTENTS

# INTRODUCTION

Each of us is unique, which is why the most effective diet plan for any woman is one that is tailor-made to meet her personal needs. If you are to maximize your health and well-being you have to know how best to do this at your particular stage in life and in your particular situation.

The good news is that working out a health-care plan that matches the complexity of your life is not impossible. With a guide to follow and a mindset geared towards success, you'll be on your way to a healthier you in no time.

As we age, it becomes more imperative that we obtain as much information as possible in order to embrace a lifestyle that encourages good health and helps create a sense of well-being. Women over 50 have shown a great interest in gaining as much information as possible in order to sustain their current health and to make sensible choices about their lifestyles and behaviors. This natural curiosity helps us to acquire new eating habits and modify our exercise routines in order to ensure a more satisfying and longer life. We turn our attention to medical research on nutrition and nutritional needs in order to learn as much as possible about our own health and how to care for our bodies. The results are finally provided, it often seems as though the medical community is playing a game of Russian roulette and the findings seem to change like the seasons.

It can be frustrating when things you thought were right are turned inside-out as new findings come to light. One moment you are told to eat more carbohydrates, and the next you're told that carbohydrates are the cause of your excess weight. Knowledge from medical research usually builds up only slowly, and sometimes it changes completely as more information becomes available.

What you'll find here is information on how to create and maintain a healthy lifestyle. The keto diet has been around for a very long time and has been proved to be one of the most comprehensive eating plans to not only help you lose unwanted pounds but to help you create a life-long way of eating that will ensure the best of health for years to come.

## THE SCIENCE BEHIND THE DIET

One of the toughest things to do when starting any diet is choosing which diet to start. There are literally hundreds of diets to choose from at any given time. Many of these diets make promises of all kinds including effortless weight loss without sacrifice and without hunger. They offer quick results with minimal effort. They share their gimmicks, tricks, and hooks to get you excited enough to begin, but fall short of explaining the science behind their promises. Usually, because there is no science. Just fad after fad that someone has thought up to make money. You know how their story ends. You start, you fall, and you fail. And you end up right back where you started, very often, having added a couple of extra pounds to top it all off.

The keto diet is much more than a fad diet; it will actually teach you a new way of eating that is not just for the time being, but forever. The science is flawless, the results have proven time and time again. It is a completely new way of eating that is not just for the moment—but is sustainable for a lifetime. You will be training your body to treat food in a whole new way.

The keto diet was originally developed by researchers and doctors for children with epilepsy. Studies proved that this special high-fat, very low-carb and protein plan helped to control, if not eliminate, seizures in children and adults with this debilitating disease. Over the course of the studies, it was noted that the patient's weights were affected in a positive way.

Let's take a moment and reflect on what we are actually talking about here. The word "diet" has such a negative connotation in today's world. It brings to mind images of celery sticks and carrots, starvation, and a never-ending struggle with will power. It implies that someone has issues with eating habits, most specifically, overeating. But that's not what the word should mean to us. If you check a dictionary, you'll find that the word diet is simply a reference to the type of foods that a person, community, or animal habitually eats.

Let's begin by embracing the idea that the keto diet is not really a "diet" at all, but merely a habitual way of eating to create a healthy body. We aren't going to "restrict" our foods, we may eliminate some, and we may control portions on others, but we will not think of our new-way-of-eating as depriving ourselves—but instead, that we are creating a pathway to a healthier and happy body, and consider this new-way-of-eating as the right path to lead us towards that goal.

# WHAT IS KETO DIET?

As you'd probably already know, the ketogenic diet is a low-carb diet where you eliminate or minimize carbohydrate intake. Proteins and fats replace the extra carbs while you cut back on pastries and sugar.

## HOW DOES IT WORK?

See, when you consume less than 50 grams of carbs per day, your body starts to run out of blood sugar (which is used as fuel to provide your body quick energy). Once there are no sugar reserves left, your body will start to utilize fat and protein for energy. This entire process is known as ketosis, and this is exactly what helps you lose weight.

## GETTING INTO KETOSIS

The process of ketosis is named after the byproduct, which is produced along with energy when a fat molecule is broken down. It is known as a ketone. When a person switches to the ketogenic approach, his body too switches to ketosis to meet the energy needs. It metabolizes fats and produces more ketones than usual. These ketones are mainly responsible for decreasing the oxidative stress of the body and detoxify the mind and body. Thus, ketosis works in three ways: by reducing the carb intake, it controls weight gain; then it provides energy through the breakdown of fats, which is more lasting; and finally, through the release of ketones, it regulates improved metabolism.

## SIGNS THAT YOU ARE IN KETOSIS

Since the human body heavily depends on carbs, it always takes time for the body to adapt to the new ketogenic lifestyle. It's like changing the fuel of a machine when the body is switched to the ketogenic diet; it shows some different signs than usual, which are as follows:

**Increased Urination**

Ketones are normally known as a diuretic, which means that they help remove the extra water out of the body through increased urination. So high levels of ketones mean more urination than normal. Due to ketosis, more acetoacetate is released about three times faster than usual, which is excreted along with urine, and its release then causes more urination.

### Dry Mouth

It is obvious that more urination means the loss of high amounts of water, which causes dehydration as more water is released out of the body due to ketosis. Along with those fluids, many metabolites and electrolytes are also excreted out of the body. Therefore, it is always recommended to increase the water consumption on a ketogenic diet, along with a good intake of electrolytes, to maintain the water levels of the body.

### Bad Breath

A ketone, which is known as acetone, is released through our breath. This ketone has a distinct smell, and it takes some time to go away. Due to ketosis, a high number of acetones are released through the breath, which causes bad breath.

### Reduced Appetite and Lasting Energy

This is the clearest sign of ketosis. Since fat molecules are high-energy macronutrients, each molecule is broken down to produce three times more energy than a carb molecule. Therefore, a person feels more energized round the clock.

## WHY SHOULD YOU SWITCH TO KETO?

Once you start to hit 50, you likely don't indulge in strenuous activities anymore, so your body will need fewer calories to function. This is when you should start eliminating added sugars from your diet. Plus, a low-carb diet that is rich in healthy vegetables and meat will prove to be far better for people suffering from insulin insensitivity and your overall health. Hence, start reading food labels more often and opt for healthier options.

Compared to other diets, keto has a better chance of helping you lose weight more quickly. The diet is also incredibly popular as you're not encouraged to starve yourself. It would help if you worked towards a more high-fat and protein diet, which isn't as difficult as counting calories. A recent study from the Hebrew University of Jerusalem has indicated how eating a diet rich in healthy fats can help you lose weight in the long-term.

Therefore, the ketogenic diet prescribes the use of fat-rich substances, like all vegetable oils, nut oils, cheese, cream cheese, butter, and creams. On the other hand, it restricts the daily carb intake to only 50 grams or less. On a ketogenic diet, a person must avoid the intake of grains, legumes, starchy vegetables, high-sugar fruits, sugars, sugary beverages and drinks, and all other products containing these basic items. These ingredients must be replaced with non-starchy vegetables, sugar-free products, meat, seafood, nut-based milk and processed dairy items.

# MACRONUTRIENTS AND KETO

The food you consume provides nutrition to the body. Various types of nutrients are present in the food. They are broadly classified into macronutrients and micronutrients. Macronutrients are those nutrients required in significant quantities in the food to provide necessary energy and raw material to build different body parts. These are:

- Carbohydrates
- Proteins
- Fats

## CARBOHYDRATES

Carbohydrates are important energy sources of the body. In a Keto diet plan, you have to cut on your carbs to eliminate this energy source and compel your body to spend the already present food stores in your body. These food stores are present as fat in your body. Once your body turns to these fat deposits for energy, you start to lose weight.

Carbohydrates should not constitute more than 5–10% of your daily caloric intake.

Carbohydrates are present in a variety of foods. You should make sure that the small quota of carbohydrates you can consume comes from healthy carbohydrate sources like low-carb vegetables and fruits, e.g., broccoli, lemon, and tomatoes.

## PROTEINS

Proteins are really important because they provide subunits, which are building blocks of the body. They produce various hormones, muscles, enzymes, and other working machinery of the body. They provide energy to the body as well.

No more than 20-25% of your daily caloric intake should come from proteins. As a rule of thumb, a healthy person should consume about 0.5-0.7 grams of proteins per pound of total body weight.

Many people make a mistake in a keto diet consuming much more protein than they should. This not only puts additional strain on their kidneys, but is also very unhealthy for the digestive system.

Eat a good variety of proteins from various sources like tofu, fish, chicken, and other white meat sources, including seeds, nuts, eggs, and dairy (though you shouldn't fill your diet with cheese). Red meat like beef can be enjoyed less frequently. We also suggest you avoid processed meats, which are typically laden with artificial preservatives.

Processed meat refers to meat that's modified through a series of processes, which might include salting, smoking, canning, and, most importantly, treated with preservatives. Such variants typically include sausages, jerky, and salami. As these meats are not even considered healthy for normal diets, we suggest limiting your portions to only once or twice a week.

# FATS

In keto, fats serve as the mainstay of your diet. It seems counterintuitive to consume what you want to eliminate from your body, but that is exactly how this strategy works. But before you go about loading your body with all types of fats, keep the following things in your mind:

1. You have to cut on carbs before this high-fat diet can be of any benefit to the body.
2. Fats should take up about 70-75% of your daily caloric intake.
3. Fats are of various types, and you have to be aware of the kind of fats you should consume.

Dietary fats can be divided into two kinds: healthy and harmful. Unsaturated fats belong to the healthier group, whereas saturated and trans-unsaturated fats belong to the unhealthier category. Aside from the differences in their health effects, these fats essentially differ in terms of chemical structure and bonding.

## Saturated Fats

Saturated fats drive up cholesterol levels and contain harmful LDL cholesterol that can clog arteries anywhere in the body, especially the heart, and increase the risk of cardiovascular diseases. These fats are mainly contained in animal origin (except fish, which contains a small part). They are also present in plant-based foods, such as coconut oil. However, coconut oil contains medium-chain fatty acids, which are saturated fats different from animal origin, and therefore considered a healthy food.

## Trans Fats

Trans fats, or trans-fatty acids, are a particular form of unsaturated fat. These unhealthy fats are manufactured through a partial hydrogenation food process. Moreover, some studies differentiate the health risks of those obtained industrially or transformed by cooking, from those naturally present in food (for example, vaccenic acid); the latter would be harmless or even beneficial to health.

The industrial foods that contain these hydrogenated fats are mainly: fried foods (especially French fries), margarine, microwave popcorn, brioche, sweet snacks, and pretzels.

While these foods may taste good, they're an unhealthy kind of fat and should be avoided.

Trans fats are known to increase unhealthy cholesterol levels in the blood, thus increasing the risks of cardiovascular disease.

## Unsaturated Fats

These "good fats" contain healthy cholesterol. Unsaturated fats can most commonly be found in nuts, veggies, and fish. These fats keep your heart healthy and are a good substitution for saturated fats.

# AGING AND NUTRITIONAL NEEDS

At any age, proper nutrition is incredibly important, but as we age, our bodies are going through some major changes. To help with these changes, it will be essential to make certain adjustments to our routines and nutrition. The vital factor to remember is that it is never too late to start taking care of yourself. When you neglect your health after the age of fifty, the effects may become more noticeable than ever before. So, how exactly does age affect our nutritional needs?

As we age, you can expect a number of different changes to happen in your body, including thinner skin, loss of muscle, and less stomach acid. When these things happen, this can, unfortunately, make you more prone to nutrient deficiencies and overall quality of life. This is where the Ketogenic Diet comes in handy! By eating a variety of foods and incorporating the proper supplements, you will be able to meet your nutrient needs with no issues! Below, you will find some of the effects of aging and how to help the issue.

## Less Calories—More Nutrients

On a general basis, an individual's daily calorie count will depend on a number of factors, including activity level, muscle mass, weight, and height. In order to maintain or lose weight, we will need to begin lowering the number of calories we take in. Generally, older adults tend to exercise and move less compared to younger individuals.

While consuming fewer calories, it is important to continue getting higher levels of nutrients. For this reason, it is highly suggested to consume a variety of foods such as low-carb vegetables and lean meats to help get the proper nutrients and fight against any nutrient deficiencies. The nutrients you will want to focus on include vitamin B12, calcium, and vitamin D, Magnesium, Potassium, Omega-3, fatty acids, and Iron.

## Benefits of Fiber

While many people do not like to discuss this, constipation is a prevalent health issue for individuals over the age of 50. In fact, women over the age of 65 are two to three times more likely to experience constipation! This may be due to the fact that people over the age of 50 generally move less and are more likely to be taking a medication that has constipation as an unfortunate side effect.

To help relieve constipation, you will want to make sure you are getting enough fiber. When you eat more fiber, it is able to pass through your gut, undigested, and help regulate bowel movements and form stool. As an added benefit, high-fiber diets may also be able to prevent diverticular disease. Diverticular disease is a condition where small pouches build along the wall of the colon and become inflamed.

## Focus on Protein

As we age, it is very common to lose both strength and muscle. In fact, on average, an adult will lose anywhere between 3-8% of their muscle mass per decade after the age of 30. When we lose muscle mass, it could lead to poor health, fractures, and weakness among the elderly population. By eating more protein, you can help fight sarcopenia and maintain your muscle mass.

## Vitamin B12

As mentioned earlier, keeping up with proper nutrients is going to be vital for your health. One of the vitamins you will want to focus on is Vitamin B12. This is a water-soluble vitamin that is in charge of making red blood cells and keeping your brain healthy. Unfortunately, it is estimated that anywhere from 1-30% of individuals over the age of 50 have a lowered ability to absorb this vitamin from their diet.

One of the main reasons individuals over the age of 50 have difficulty absorbing vitamin B12 may be due to the fact that they have reduced stomach acid reduction. Vitamin B12 is bound to proteins. In order for your body to use this vitamin, the stomach acid separates it from the protein and becomes absorbed. To benefit your new diet, you will want to consider taking a supplement of vitamin B12 or consuming foods that are fortified with the vitamin.

## Vitamin D and Calcium

When it comes to bone health, calcium and vitamin D are going to be very important. While calcium is in charge of maintaining and building healthy bones, it depends on vitamin D to help the body absorb the calcium in the first place! Unfortunately, adults have a harder time absorbing calcium in their diets. This may be due to the fact that the gut absorbs less calcium as we age. However, the main culprit of a reduction in calcium is typically due to a vitamin D deficiency. As you can tell, they work hand in hand!

The reason we may experience a vitamin D deficiency is due to thinning skin. Generally, our body makes vitamin D from the cholesterol in the skin when it is exposed to sunlight. As the skin becomes thinner, it reduces the ability to make vitamin D and, in turn, reduces the ability to get enough calcium. When these two things happen, it increases the risk of fractures and bone loss.

To help counter this aging effect, you will want to make sure you are getting enough vitamin D and calcium in your diet. Some accessible sources will be dairy products, leafy vegetables, and dark greens. As far as Vitamin D goes, you will want to include a variety of fish or even a Vitamin D supplement such as cod liver oil.

## Dehydration

On the Ketogenic Diet or not, staying hydrated is important at any age. In fact, water makes up about 60% of our bodies! Whether you are 20, 30, or 50, the body still continually loses water through urine and sweat. As we age, it makes us more prone to dehydration.

When we become dehydrated, the water detects the thirst through receptors found all throughout the body and the brain. As we age, the receptors become less sensitive, making it hard to distinguish the thirst in the first place. On top of this, our kidneys are there to help converse water, but they also lose function with age.

Unfortunately, the consequences of dehydration are pretty harsh for the older population. When you are dehydrated long-term, this could reduce your ability to absorb medication and could worsen any medical condition. For this reason, it will be vital you keep up with your intake of water. I suggest trying a water challenge with friends and family or try having a glass of water with each meal you have.

## Appetite

The last topic we will tackle is the decrease in appetite. While this may seem like a benefit, a lack of eating could lead to a number of different nutritional deficiencies and unwanted weight loss. Poor appetite is most commonly linked to poor health.

It is believed that some of the significant factors behind appetite loss could be due to changes in smell, taste, and hormones. Generally, older adults who have lower levels of hunger have higher levels of fullness hormones. When this happens, it causes individuals to be less hungry overall. As we age, the changes in smell and taste can also make food seem less appealing.

If you find this happens to you, you may want to establish a healthy habit of snacking. When you snack, try to reach for keto-friendly foods such as eggs, and almonds to help put the nutrients back into your diet. If you are aware of this issue, it is something you can get a grasp on before it becomes a real problem.

# IMPORTANT HEALTH TIPS AFTER 50

Nobody told you that life was going to be this way! But don't worry. There's still plenty of time to make amendments and take care of your health. Here are a couple of tips that will allow you to lead a healthier life in your fifties:

## START BUILDING ON IMMUNITY

Every day, our body is exposed to free radicals and toxins from the environment. The added stress of work and family problems doesn't make it any easier for us. To combat this, you must start consuming healthy veggies that contain plenty of antioxidants and build a healthier immune system.

This helps ward off unwanted illnesses and diseases, allowing you to maintain good health.

Adding healthier veggies to your keto diet will help you obtain various minerals, vitamins, and antioxidants.

## CONSIDER QUITTING SMOKING

It's never too late to try to quit smoking, even if you are in your fifties. Once a smoker begins to quit, the body quickly starts to heal the previous damages caused by smoking.

Once you start quitting, you'll notice how you'll be able to breathe easier while acquiring a better sense of smell and taste. Over a period of time, eliminating the habit of smoking can greatly reduce the risks of high blood pressure, strokes, and heart attack. Please note how these diseases are much more common among people in the fifties and above than in younger people.

Not to mention, quitting smoking will help you stay more active and enjoy better health with your friends and family.

## STAY SOCIAL

Aging can be a daunting process, and trying to get through it all on your own isn't particularly helpful. We recommend you to stay in touch with friends and family or become a part of a local community club or network. Some older people find it comforting to get an emotional support animal.

Being surrounded by people you love will give you a sense of belonging and will improve your mood. It'll also keep your mind and memory sharp as you engage in different conversations.

# HEALTH SCREENINGS YOU SHOULD GET AFTER YOUR FIFTIES

Don't let the joy of these years be robbed away from you because of poor health. Getting simple tests done can go a long way in identifying any potential health problems that you may have. Here is a list of health screenings you should get done:

## Check Your Blood Pressure

Your blood pressure is a reliable indicator of your heart health. In simple words, blood pressure is a measure of how fast blood travels through the artery walls. Very high or even very low blood pressure can be a sign of an underlying problem. Once you reach your 50s, you should have your blood pressure checked more often.

## EKG

The EKG reveals your heart health and activity. Short for electrocardiogram, the EKG helps identify problems in the heart. The process works by highlighting any rhythm problems that may be in the heart, such as poor heart muscles, improper blood flow, or any other form of abnormality. Getting an EKG is also a predictive measure for understanding the chances of a heart attack. Since people starting their fifties are at greater risk of getting a heart attack, you should get yourself checked more often.

## Mammogram

Mammograms help rule out the risks of breast cancer. Women who enter their fifties should ideally get a mammogram every two years. If you have a family history, getting one becomes especially important.

## Blood Sugar Levels

If you're somebody who used to grab a fast food meal every once in a while before you switched to keto, then you should definitely check your blood sugar levels more carefully. Blood sugar levels indicate whether or not you have diabetes. And you know how the saying goes, "prevention is better than cure." It's best to clear these possibilities out of the way sooner than later.

## Check for Osteoporosis

Unfortunately, as you grow older, you also become susceptible to a number of bone diseases. Osteoporosis is a bone-related condition in which bones begin to lose mass, becoming frail and weak. Owing to this, seniors become more prone to fractures. This can make even the smallest of falls detrimental to your health.

## Annual Physical Exam

Your insurance must be providing coverage for your annual physical exam. So, there's no reason why you should not take advantage of it. This checkup helps identify the state of your health. You'll probably be surprised by how much doctors can tell from a single blood test.

## Eye Exam

As you start to aging, you'll notice how your eyesight will start to deteriorate. It's quite likely that vision is not as sharp as it used to be. Ideally, you should have gotten your first eye exam during your 40s, but it isn't too late. Get one as soon as possible to prevent symptoms from escalating.

## Be Wary Of Any Weird Moles

While skin cancer can become a problem at any age, older adults should pay closer attention to any moles or unusual skin tags in their bodies. While most cancers can be easily treated, melanoma can be particularly quite dangerous. If you have noticed any recent moles in your body that have changed in color, size, or shape, make sure to visit the dermatologist.

## Check Your Cholesterol Levels

High cholesterol levels can be dangerous to your health and can be an indicator of many diseases. Things become more complicated for conditions that don't show particular symptoms. Your total cholesterol levels should be below 200 mg per deciliter just to be on the safe side. Your doctor will take a simple blood test and will give you a couple of guidelines with the results. In case there is something to be worried about, you should make serious dietary and lifestyle changes.

# KETOGENIC DIET AND MENOPAUSE

There comes an age in a woman's life where her menstrual cycle will finally end. This is when your ovaries stop releasing eggs, better known as ovulation, and therefore menstruation ends. This condition is generally observed in women above the age of 50. There is no defined age that shows when a woman can expect menopause.

There are times where women may experience menopause prematurely as well. This happens if a woman has undergone surgeries like hysterectomy (surgery that involves the removal of ovaries). It can also happen from any injuries that may have caused damage to the ovaries. If this happens before the age of 50, it is classified as premature menopause.

Menopause, as harmless as it sounds, can be quite a troubling phase for women. The hot flashes you experience will keep you up at night, with an elevated heartbeat. The constant feeling of being irritated and a clear downfall in your sex life can contribute greatly towards you feeling more and more grumpy.

Menopause takes a toll on your hormonal balance and the newly developed imbalance then pushes your body to gain massive weight, experience mood swings like never before, and a libido that is crashing faster than you can imagine.

If you think this is bad, here are some other issues that menopause can lead to:

- Chronic stress
- Anxiety
- Insulin spike
- Type 2 diabetes
- Heart diseases
- Polycystic Ovarian Syndrome (PCOS)

The overall picture, then, is grim! Fortunately, a difference in lifestyle and a carefully thought-out diet plan can change all that for you. I am not saying it happens overnight or within a week, but the profound impacts are felt rather quickly. In the longer run, keto will rescue you and your body from impending doom and allow you to lead a life without worrying about keeping a glucose monitor or any of the typical health-related equipment near you.

The keto diet, while there are many classes of it, helps your hormones be balanced. This means that you do not have to worry about insulin or any other hormones, hence minimizing the hot flashes and other symptoms. Even if they occur, they will be minor and far less painful.

Moreover, the keto diet jump-starts your sex drive. The fat-rich diet improves fat-soluble vitamin absorption. Not to forget, it especially helps with vitamin D, a vital micronutrient that goes missing with age. All in all, this provides all the drive you need to have intimate moments even in your fifties.

## Heart Diseases

Keto diets help women over 50 to shed those extra pounds. Reducing any amount of weight greatly reduces the chances of a heart attack or any other heart complications. Through a carefully selected diet routine, not only are you losing weight and enjoying scrumptious meals, but you are significantly boosting your heart's health and reviving yourself from the otherwise dull state that you may have been in before.

## Diabetes Control

Needless to say, the careful selection of ingredients, when cooked together, provide nutrition that is free from any processed or harmful contents such as sugar. Add this to the fact that keto automatically controls your insulin levels. The result is a glucose level that is always under control and continued control would lead to a day where you will say goodbye to the medications you might be taking for diabetes.

## And so Much More!

By taking up the challenge and adapting the keto way, you are ensuring yourself one of the safest journeys into the older years, if not the safest of the lot. Sure, there will be days where you may miss a type of food or two, but that craving will be overshadowed by the benefits the keto diet will bring you.

With the help of the keto diet, you can expect a few more benefits such as:

- Improved and stable blood pressure levels
- A deeper sleep for those suffering from insomnia
- Improved kidney function
- More energy that lasts all day
- Improved bodily functions

# BREAKFAST RECIPES
## THREE CHEESE EGG MUFFINS

PREPARATION TIME: 5 MINUTES | COOKING TIME: 20 MINUTES | SERVINGS: 12

**INGREDIENTS:**

1 tablespoon butter

½ cup diced yellow onion

12 large eggs, whisked

¼ cup cooked bacon, chopped

½ cup canned coconut milk

¼ cup sliced green onion

Salt and pepper

½ cup shredded cheddar cheese

½ cup shredded Swiss cheese

¼ cup grated parmesan cheese

**DIRECTIONS:**

1. Preheat the oven to 350°F and grease the cooking spray into a muffin pan.
2. Melt the butter over moderate heat in a medium skillet.
3. Add the onions, then cook until softened for 3 to 4 minutes.
4. Divide the mix between cups of muffins.
5. Whisk the bacon, coconut milk, green onions, salt, and pepper together and then spoon into the muffin cups.
6. In a cup, mix the three kinds of cheese and scatter over the egg muffins.
7. Bake till the egg is set, for 20 to 25 minutes.

**NUTRITION:**

Calories: 150; Fat: 11.5g; Protein: 10g; Carbohydrates: 2g.

# BACON APPETIZERS

PREPARATION TIME: 15 MINUTES | COOKING TIME: 2 HOURS | SERVINGS: 6

## INGREDIENTS:

1 pack Keto crackers

¾ cup Parmesan cheese, grated

1 pound bacon, sliced thinly

## DIRECTIONS:

1. Preheat your oven to 250°F.
2. Arrange the crackers on a baking sheet.
3. Sprinkle cheese on top of each cracker.
4. Wrap each cracker with the bacon.
5. Bake in the oven for 2 hours.

## NUTRITION:

Calories: 440; Fat: 33.4g; Protein: 29.4g; Carbohydrates: 3.7g.

# MORNING COFFEE WITH CREAM

PREPARATION TIME: O MINUTES  |  COOKING TIME: 5 MINUTES  |  SERVINGS: 1

**INGREDIENTS:**

¾ cup coffee

¼ cup whipping cream

**DIRECTIONS:**

1. Make your favorite coffee.
2. Pour the heavy cream in a small saucepan and heat slowly until you get a frothy texture.
3. Pour the hot cream in a big cup, add coffee and enjoy your morning drink.

**NUTRITION:**

Calories: 202; Fat: 21g; Protein: 2g; Carbohydrates: 2g.

# ANTIPASTI SKEWERS

PREPARATION TIME: 10 MINUTES  |  COOKING TIME: 0 MINUTE  |  SERVINGS: 6

**INGREDIENTS:**

6 small mozzarella balls

1 tablespoon olive oil

Salt to taste

1/8 teaspoon dried oregano

2 roasted yellow peppers, sliced into strips and rolled

6 cherry tomatoes

6 green olives, pitted

6 Kalamata olives, pitted

2 artichoke hearts, sliced into wedges

6 slices bacon, rolled

6 leaves fresh basil

**DIRECTIONS:**

1. Toss the mozzarella balls in olive oil.
2. Season with salt and oregano.
3. Thread the mozzarella balls and the rest of the ingredients into skewers.
4. Serve on a platter.

**NUTRITION:**

Calories: 180; Fat: 11.8g; Protein: 9.2g; Carbohydrates: 11.7g.

# JALAPENO POPPERS

PREPARATION TIME: 30 MINUTES  |  COOKING TIME: 60 MINUTES  |  SERVINGS: 10

**INGREDIENTS:**

5 fresh jalapenos, sliced and seeded

4 ounces package cream cheese

¼ pound bacon, sliced in half

**DIRECTIONS:**

1. Preheat your oven to 275°F.
2. Place a wire rack over your baking sheet.
3. Stuff each jalapeno with cream cheese and wrap in bacon.
4. Secure with a toothpick.
5. Place on the baking sheet.
6. Bake for 1 hour and 15 minutes.

**NUTRITION:**

Calories: 103; Fat: 4.1g; Protein: 5.2g; Carbohydrates: 0.9g.

# EGGS BENEDICT DEVILED EGGS

PREPARATION TIME: 15 MINUTES | COOKING TIME: 25 MINUTES | SERVINGS: 16

## INGREDIENTS:

8 hardboiled eggs, sliced in half

1 tablespoon lemon juice

½ teaspoon mustard powder

1 pack Hollandaise sauce mix, prepared according to direction on the packaging

1 pound asparagus, trimmed and steamed

4 ounces bacon, cooked and chopped

## DIRECTIONS:

1. Scoop out the egg yolks.
2. Mix the egg yolks with lemon juice, mustard powder and 1/3 cup of the Hollandaise sauce.
3. Spoon the egg yolk mixture into each of the egg whites.
4. Arrange the asparagus spears on a serving plate.
5. Top with the deviled eggs.
6. Sprinkle remaining sauce and bacon on top.

## NUTRITION:

Calories: 80; Fat: 5.3g; Protein: 6.2g; Carbohydrates: 2.1g.

# KETO BREAKFAST CHEESECAKE

PREPARATION TIME: 20 MINUTES | COOKING TIME: 45 MINUTES | SERVINGS: 24 MINI CHEESECAKES

## INGREDIENTS:

**Toppings:**

¼ cup mixed berries for each cheesecake, frozen and thawed

**For filling:**

½ teaspoon vanilla extract

½ teaspoon almond extract

¾ cup sweetener

6 eggs

8 ounces cream cheese

16 ounces cottage cheese

**For crust:**

4 tablespoons salted butter

2 tablespoons sweetener

2 cups almonds, whole

## DIRECTIONS:

1. Preheat oven to around 350°F.

2. Pulse almonds in a food processor, then add in butter and sweetener.

3. Pulse until all the ingredients mix well and a coarse dough forms.

4. Coat twelve silicone muffin pans using foil or paper liners.

5. Divide the batter evenly between the muffin pans, then press into the bottom part until it forms a crust and bakes for about 8 minutes.

6. In the meantime, mix the cream cheese and cottage cheese in a food processor, then pulse until the mixture is smooth.

7. Put in the extracts and sweetener, then combine until well mixed.

8. Add in eggs and pulse again until it becomes smooth; you might need to scrape down the mixture from the sides of the processor. Share the batter equally between the muffin pans, then bake for around 30-40 minutes until the middle is not wobbly when you shake the muffin pan lightly.

9. Put aside until cooled completely, then put in the refrigerator for about 2 hours and top with frozen and thawed berries.

## NUTRITION:

Calories: 152; Fat: 12g; Protein: 6g; Carbohydrates: 3g.

# EGG-CRUST PIZZA

PREPARATION TIME: 5 MINUTES | COOKING TIME: 15 MINUTES | SERVINGS: 1-2

## INGREDIENTS:

¼ teaspoon dried oregano to taste

½ teaspoon spike seasoning to taste

1 ounce mozzarella, chopped into small cubes

6-8 sliced thinly black olives

6 slices turkey pepperoni, sliced in half

4-5 thinly sliced small grape tomatoes

2 eggs, beaten well

1-2 teaspoons olive oil

## DIRECTIONS:

1.  Preheat the broiler in an oven, then beat the eggs well in a small bowl. Cut the pepperoni and tomatoes in slices, then cut the mozzarella cheese into cubes.

2.  Put some olive oil in a skillet over medium heat, then heat the pan for around one minute until it begins to get hot. Add in eggs and season with oregano and spike seasoning, then cook for around 2 minutes until the eggs begin to set at the bottom.

3.  Drizzle half of the mozzarella, olives, pepperoni, and tomatoes on the eggs, followed by another layer of the remaining half of the above ingredients. Ensure that there is a lot of cheese on the topmost layers. Cover the skillet using a lid and cook until the cheese begins to melt and the eggs are set, for around 3-4 minutes.

4.  Place the pan under the preheated broiler and cook until the top has browned and the cheese has melted nicely for around 2-3 minutes. Serve immediately.

## NUTRITION:

Calories: 363; Fat: 24.1g; Protein: 19.25g; Carbohydrates: 20.8g.

# BASIC OPIE ROLLS

PREPARATION TIME: 20 MINUTES  |  COOKING TIME: 35 MINUTES  |  SERVINGS: 12 ROLLS

## INGREDIENTS:

1/8 teaspoon salt

1/8 teaspoon cream of tartar

3 ounces cream cheese

3 large eggs

## DIRECTIONS:

1. Preheat the oven to about 300°F, then separate the egg whites from egg yolks and place both eggs in different bowls. Using an electric mixer, beat the egg whites well until the mixture is very bubbly, then add in the cream of tartar and mix again until it forms a stiff peak.

2. In the bowl with the egg yolks, put in 3 ounces of cubed cheese and salt. Mix well until the mixture has doubled in size and is pale yellow. Put the egg white mixture into the egg yolk mixture, then fold the mixture gently together.

3. Spray some oil on the cookie sheet coated with some parchment paper, then add dollops of the batter and bake for around 30 minutes.

4. You will know they are ready when the upper part of the rolls are firm and golden. Leave them to cool for a few minutes on a wire rack. Enjoy with some coffee.

## NUTRITION:

Calories: 43; Fat: 3.7g; Protein: 2.1g; Carbohydrates: 0.3g.

# CELERY JUICE

PREPARATION TIME: 10 MINUTES | COOKING TIME: 0 MINUTES | SERVINGS: 2

**INGREDIENTS:**

8 celery stalks with leaves

2 tablespoons fresh ginger, peeled

1 lemon, peeled

½ cup of filtered water

Pinch of salt

**DIRECTIONS:**

1. Place all the ingredients in a blender and pulse until well combined.

2. Through a fine mesh strainer, strain the juice and transfer it into 2 glasses.

3. Serve immediately.

**NUTRITION:**

Calories: 32; Fat: 1.1g; Protein: 1.2g; Carbohydrates: 1.3g.

# GRAPEFRUIT & CELERY BLAST

PREPARATION TIME: 10 MINUTES | COOKING TIME: 0 MINUTES | SERVINGS: 1

**INGREDIENTS:**

1 grapefruit, peeled

2 stalks of celery

2 ounces kale

½ teaspoon matcha powder

**DIRECTIONS:**

1. Place ingredients into a blender with water to cover them and blitz until smooth.

**NUTRITION:**

Calories: 129; Fat: 2.1g; Protein: 1.2g; Carbohydrates: 12.1g.

# LEMONY GREEN JUICE

PREPARATION TIME: 10 MINUTES | COOKING TIME: 0 MINUTES | SERVINGS: 2

**INGREDIENTS:**

2 large green apples, cored and sliced

4 cups fresh kale leaves

4 tablespoons fresh parsley leaves

1 tablespoon fresh ginger, peeled

1 lemon, peeled

½ cup of filtered water

Pinch of salt

**DIRECTIONS:**

1. Place all the ingredients in a blender and pulse until well combined.

2. Through a fine mesh strainer, strain the juice and transfer it into 2 glasses.

3. Serve immediately.

**NUTRITION:**

Calories: 196; Fat: 1.1g; Protein: 1.5g; Carbohydrates: 1.6g.

# CHOCOLATE SEA SALT SMOOTHIE

PREPARATION TIME: 15 MINUTES  |  COOKING TIME: 0 MINUTES  |  SERVINGS: 2

**INGREDIENTS:**

1 avocado

2 cups almond milk

1 tablespoon tahini

¼ cup of cocoa powder

1 scoop Keto chocolate base

**DIRECTIONS:**

1. Combine all the fixing in a high-speed blender. Add ice and serve!

**NUTRITION:**

Calories: 235; Fat: 20g; Protein: 5.5g; Carbohydrates: 11.25g.

# ORANGE & CELERY CRUSH

PREPARATION TIME: 10 MINUTES | COOKING TIME: 0 MINUTES | SERVINGS: 1

## INGREDIENTS:

1 carrot, peeled

Stalks of celery

1 orange, peeled

½ teaspoon matcha powder

Juice of 1 lime

## DIRECTIONS:

1. Place ingredients into a blender with enough water to cover them and blitz until smooth.

## NUTRITION:

Calories: 150; Fat: 2.1g; Protein: 1.4g; Carbohydrates: 11.2g.

# CREAMY STRAWBERRY & CHERRY SMOOTHIE

PREPARATION TIME: 10 MINUTES  |  COOKING TIME: 0 MINUTES  |  SERVINGS: 1

## INGREDIENTS:

3 ½ ounces strawberries

1 ounce of frozen pitted cherries

1 tablespoon Greek yogurt

1 ounce of unsweetened soya milk

## DIRECTIONS:

1. Place the ingredients into a blender then process until smooth.

2. Serve and enjoy.

## NUTRITION:

Calories: 203; Fat: 3.1g; Protein: 1.7g; Carbohydrates: 9g

# ROSEMARY CHEESE CHIPS WITH GUACAMOLE

PREPARATION TIME: 10 MINUTES | COOKING TIME: 20 MINUTES | SERVINGS: 4

## INGREDIENTS:

1 tablespoon rosemary

1 cup Grana Padano, grated

¼ teaspoon sweet paprika

¼ teaspoon garlic powder

2 avocados, pitted and scooped

1 tomato, chopped

## DIRECTIONS:

1. Preheat oven to 350°F and line a baking sheet with parchment paper. Mix Grana Padano cheese, paprika, rosemary, and garlic powder evenly.

2. Spoon 6-8 teaspoons on the baking sheet creating spaces between each mound.

3. Flatten mounds. Bake for 5 minutes, cool, and remove to a plate. To make the guacamole, mash avocado, with a fork in a bowl, add in tomato, and continue to mash until mostly smooth. Season with salt.

4. Serve crackers with guacamole.

## NUTRITION:

Calories: 229; Fat: 20g; Protein: 10g; Carbohydrates: 2,6g

# BAKED CHORIZO WITH COTTAGE CHEESE

PREPARATION TIME: 10 MINUTES | COOKING TIME: 30 MINUTES | SERVINGS: 6

**INGREDIENTS:**

7 ounces Spanish chorizo, sliced

4 ounces cottage cheese, pureed

¼ cup chopped parsley

**DIRECTIONS:**

1. Preheat the oven to 325°F. Line a baking dish with waxed paper. Bake the chorizo for minutes until crispy. Remove from the oven and let cool.

2. Arrange on a Serves platter. Top each slice with cottage cheese and parsley.

**NUTRITION:**

Calories: 172; Fat: 13g; Protein: 5g; Carbohydrates: 0.52g.

# CRISPY CHORIZO WITH CHEESY TOPPING

PREPARATION TIME: 10 MINUTES  |  COOKING TIME: 30 MINUTES  |  SERVINGS: 6

**INGREDIENTS:**

7 ounces Spanish chorizo, sliced

4 ounces cream cheese

¼ cup chopped parsley

**DIRECTIONS:**

1.  Preheat oven to 325°F. Line a baking dish with waxed paper. Bake chorizo for minutes until crispy. Remove and let cool.

2.  Arrange on a serving platter. Top with cream cheese.

3.  Serve sprinkled with parsley.

**NUTRITION:**

Calories: 172; Fat: 13g; Protein: 5g; Carbohydrates: 3.3g.

# GOLDEN CHEESE CRISPS

PREPARATION TIME: 10 MINUTES  |  COOKING TIME: 10 MINUTES  |  SERVINGS: 4

**INGREDIENTS:**

1 cup Edam cheese

1 cup provolone cheese

1/3 teaspoon dried oregano

1/3 teaspoon dried rosemary

½ teaspoon garlic powder

1/3 teaspoon dried basil

**DIRECTIONS:**

1.  Preheat your oven to 390°F.

2.  In a small bowl mix the dried oregano, rosemary, basil, and garlic powder. Set aside. Combine the Edam cheese and provolone cheese in another medium bowl.

3.  Line a large baking dish with parchment paper, place tablespoon-sized stacks of the cheese mixture on the baking dish. Sprinkle with the dry seasonings mixture and bake for 6-7 minutes.

4.  Let cool for a few minutes and enjoy.

**NUTRITION:**

Calories: 296; Fat: 22.7g; Protein: 22g; Carbohydrates: 1.8g.

# MINTY ZUCCHINIS

PREPARATION TIME: 10 MINUTES | COOKING TIME: 15 MINUTES | SERVINGS: 4

## INGREDIENTS:

1 pound zucchinis, sliced

1 tablespoon olive oil

2 garlic cloves, minced

1 tablespoon mint, chopped

pinch of salt and black pepper

¼ cup veggie stock

## DIRECTIONS:

1. Heat up a pan with the oil over medium-high heat, add the garlic and sauté for 2 minutes.
2. Add the zucchinis and the other ingredients, toss, cook everything for 10 minutes more, divide between plates and serve.

## NUTRITION:

Calories: 70; Fat: 1g; Protein: 6g; Carbohydrates: 0.5g.

# CHEDDAR CAULIFLOWER BITES

PREPARATION TIME: 10 MINUTES  |  COOKING TIME: 25 MINUTES  |  SERVINGS: 8

## INGREDIENTS:

1 pound cauliflower florets

1 teaspoon sweet paprika

A pinch of salt and black pepper

2 eggs, whisked

1 cup coconut flour

Cooking spray

1 cup cheddar cheese, grated

## DIRECTIONS:

1. In a bowl, mix the flour with salt, pepper, cheese, and paprika and stir.
2. Put the eggs in a separate bowl.
3. Dredge the cauliflower florets in the eggs and then in the cheese mix, arrange them on a baking sheet lined with parchment paper and bake at 430°F for 25 minutes.
4. Serve as a snack.

## NUTRITION:

Calories: 163; Fat: 12g; Protein: 7g; Carbohydrates: 2g.

# MINI SALMON BITES

PREPARATION TIME: 10 MINUTES  |  COOKING TIME: 0 MINUTES  |  SERVINGS: 10

## INGREDIENTS:

8 ounces cream cheese, softened

4 ounces salmon fillets, chopped

2 medium scallions, thinly sliced

Bagel seasoning, as required

## DIRECTIONS:

1. In a bowl, add the cream cheese and beat until fluffy.

2. Add the salmon, and scallions and beat until well combined.

3. Make bite-sized balls from the mixture and lightly coat with the bagel seasoning.

4. Arrange the balls onto 2 parchment-lined baking sheets and refrigerate for about 2-3 hours before serving.

5. Enjoy!

## NUTRITION:

Calories: 94; Fat: 8.4g; Protein: 3.8g; Carbohydrates: 0.8g.

# DELIGHTFUL CAULIFLOWER POPPERS

PREPARATION TIME: 15 MINUTES  |  COOKING TIME: 30 MINUTES  |  SERVINGS: 4

**INGREDIENTS:**

4 cup cauliflower florets

2 teaspoon olive oil

¼ teaspoon chili powder

Salt and freshly ground black pepper, to taste

**DIRECTIONS:**

1.  Preheat the oven to 450°F. Grease a roasting pan.

2.  In a bowl, add all ingredients and toss to coat well.

3.  Transfer the cauliflower mixture into a prepared roasting pan and spread in an even layer.

4.  Roast for about 25-30 minutes.

5.  Serve warm.

**NUTRITION:**

Calories: 46; Fat: 2.5g; Protein: 2g; Carbohydrates: 5.4g.

# COCONUT CRAB CAKES

PREPARATION TIME: 20 MINUTES | COOKING TIME: 25 MINUTES | SERVINGS: 4

## INGREDIENTS:

1 tablespoon minced garlic

2 pasteurized eggs

2 teaspoons coconut oil

¾ cup coconut flakes

¾ cup chopped spinach

¼ pound crabmeat

¼ cup chopped leek

½ cup extra virgin olive oil

½ teaspoon pepper

¼ onion diced

Salt

## DIRECTIONS:

1. Pour the crabmeat in a bowl, then add in the coconut flakes and mix well.
2. Whisk eggs in a bowl, then mix in leek and spinach.
3. Season the egg mixture with pepper, two pinches of salt, and garlic.
4. Then, pour the eggs into the crab and stir well.
5. Preheat a pan, heat extra virgin olive, and fry the crab evenly from each side until golden brown. Remove from pan and serve hot.

## NUTRITION:

Calories: 254; Fat: 9.5g; Protein: 8.9g; Carbohydrates: 4.1g.

# BACON AND FETA SKEWERS

PREPARATION TIME: 15 MINUTES | COOKING TIME: 10 MINUTES | SERVINGS: 4

## INGREDIENTS:

2 pounds feta cheese, cut into 8 cubes

8 bacon slices

4 bamboo skewers, soaked

1 zucchini, cut into 8 bite-size cubes

Salt and black pepper to taste

3 tablespoons avocado oil for brushing

## DIRECTIONS:

1. Wrap each feta cube with a bacon slice.
2. Thread one wrapped feta on a skewer; add a zucchini cube, then another wrapped feta, and another zucchini.
3. Repeat the threading process with the remaining skewers.
4. Preheat a grill pan to medium heat, generously brush with the avocado oil and grill the skewer on both sides for 3 to 4 minutes per side or until the set is golden brown and the bacon cooked.
5. Serve and enjoy.

## NUTRITION:

Calories: 290; Fat: 15.1g; Protein: 11.8g; Carbohydrates: 4.1g.

# AVOCADO AND PROSCIUTTO DEVILED EGGS

PREPARATION TIME: 20 MINUTES  |  COOKING TIME: 10 MINUTES  |  SERVINGS: 4

## INGREDIENTS:

4 eggs

Ice bath

4 prosciutto slices, chopped

1 avocado, pitted and peeled

1 tablespoon mustard

1 teaspoon plain vinegar

1 tablespoon heavy cream

1 tablespoon chopped fresh cilantro

Salt and black pepper to taste

½ cup mayonnaise

1 tablespoon coconut cream

¼ teaspoon cayenne pepper

1 tablespoon avocado oil

1 tablespoon chopped fresh parsley

## DIRECTIONS:

1. Boil the eggs for 8 minutes.
2. Remove the eggs into the ice bath, sit for 3 minutes, and then peel the eggs.
3. Slice the eggs lengthwise into halves and empty the egg yolks into a bowl.
4. Arrange the egg whites on a plate with the whole side facing upwards.
5. While the eggs are cooking, heat a non-stick skillet over medium heat and cook the prosciutto for 5 to 8 minutes.
6. Remove the prosciutto onto a paper towel-lined plate to drain grease.
7. Put the avocado slices with the egg yolks and mash both ingredients with a fork until smooth.
8. Mix in the mustard, vinegar, heavy cream, cilantro, salt, and black pepper until well-blended.
9. Spoon the mixture into a piping bag and press the mixture into the egg holes until well-filled.
10. In a bowl, whisk the mayonnaise, coconut cream, cayenne pepper, and avocado oil.
11. On serving plates, spoon some of the mayonnaise sauce and slightly smear it in a circular movement. Top with the deviled eggs, scatter the prosciutto on top and garnish with the parsley.
12. Enjoy immediately.

## NUTRITION:

Calories: 265; Fat: 11.7g; Protein: 7.9g; Carbohydrates: 3.1g.

# DELECTABLE TOMATO SLICES

PREPARATION TIME: 15 MINUTES | COOKING TIME: 15 MINUTES | SERVINGS: 10

## INGREDIENTS:

½ cup mayonnaise

½ cup ricotta cheese, shredded

½ cup part-skim mozzarella cheese, shredded

½ cup Parmesan and Romano cheese blend, grated

1 teaspoon garlic, minced

1 tablespoon dried oregano, crushed

Salt, to taste

4 large tomatoes, cut each one in 5 slices

## DIRECTIONS:

1. Preheat the oven to broiler on high. Arrange a rack about 3-inch from the heating element.
2. In a bowl, add the mayonnaise, cheeses, garlic, oregano, and salt and mix until well combined and smooth.
3. Spread the cheese mixture over each tomato slice evenly.
4. Arrange the tomato slices onto a broiler pan in a single layer.
5. Broil for about 3-5 minutes or until the top becomes golden brown.
6. Remove from the oven and transfer the tomato slices onto a platter.
7. Set aside to cool slightly.
8. Serve warm.

## NUTRITION:

Calories: 110; Fat: 57.4g; Protein: 5 g; Carbohydrates: 6.7g.

# GRAIN-FREE TORTILLA CHIPS

PREPARATION TIME: 15 MINUTES  |  COOKING TIME: 16 MINUTES  |  SERVINGS: 6

## INGREDIENTS:

1 ½ cups mozzarella cheese, shredded

½ cup almond flour

1 tablespoon golden flaxseed meal

Salt and freshly ground black pepper, to taste

## DIRECTIONS:

1. Preheat the oven to 375°F. Line 2 large baking sheets with parchment paper.

2. In a microwave-safe bowl, add the cheese and microwave for about 1 minute, stirring after every 15 seconds.

3. In the bowl of melted cheese, add the almond flour, flaxseed meal, salt, and black pepper and with a fork, mix well.

4. With your hands, knead until a dough forms.

5. Make 2 equal sized balls from the dough.

6. Place 1 dough ball onto each prepared baking sheet and roll into an 8x10-inch rectangle.

7. Cut each dough rectangle into triangle-shaped chips.

8. Arrange the chips in a single layer.

9. Bake for about 10-15 minutes, flipping once halfway through.

10. Remove from oven and set aside to cool before serving.

## NUTRITION:

Calories: 80; Fat: 6.3g; Protein: 4.2g; Carbohydrates: 2.6g.

# CHEESES CHIPS

PREPARATION TIME: 15 MINUTES  |  COOKING TIME: 15 MINUTES  |  SERVINGS: 8

## INGREDIENTS:

3 tablespoons coconut flour

½ cup strong cheddar cheese, grated and divided

¼ cup Parmesan cheese, grated

2 tablespoons butter, melted

1 organic egg

1 teaspoon fresh thyme leaves, minced

## DIRECTIONS:

1.  Preheat the oven to 350°F. Line a large baking sheet with parchment paper.
2.  In a bowl, place the coconut flour, 1/4 cup of grated cheddar, Parmesan, butter, and egg and mix until well combined.
3.  Set the mixture aside for about 3-5 minutes.
4.  Make 8 equal-sized balls from the mixture.
5.  Arrange the balls onto a prepared baking sheet in a single layer about 2-inch apart.
6.  With your hands, press each ball into a little flat disc.
7.  Sprinkle each disc with the remaining cheddar, followed by thyme.
8.  Bake for about 13-15 minutes or until the edges become golden brown.
9.  Remove from the oven and let them cool completely before serving.

## NUTRITION:

Calories: 94; Fat: 7.1g; Protein: 4.2g; Carbohydrates: 3.2g.

# SNACK PARTIES TREAT

PREPARATION TIME: 10 MINUTES  |  COOKING TIME: 6 MINUTES  |  SERVINGS: 4

## INGREDIENTS:

8 bacon slices

8 mozzarella cheese sticks, frozen overnight

1 cup olive oil

## DIRECTIONS:

1. Wrap a bacon slice around each cheese stick and secure with a toothpick.

2. In a cast-iron skillet, heat the oil over medium heat and fry the mozzarella sticks in 2 batches for about 2-3 minutes or until golden brown from all sides.

3. With a slotted spoon, transfer the mozzarella sticks onto a paper towel-lined plate to drain.

4. Set aside to cool slightly.

5. Serve warm.

## NUTRITION:

Calories: 798; Fat: 76.3g; Protein: 30.1g; Carbohydrates: 2.5g.

# DELICIOUS CHICKEN WINGS

PREPARATION TIME: 10 MINUTES | COOKING TIME: 30 MINUTES | SERVINGS: 6

**INGREDIENTS:**

1 egg, beaten

1 ½ pounds chicken wings, skinless

6 tablespoons olive oil

½ cup apple cider vinegar

½ teaspoon cayenne pepper

2 garlic cloves, minced

½ teaspoon pepper

¾ teaspoon salt

**DIRECTIONS:**

1. Add all ingredients except chicken in a large bowl and mix well.
2. Add chicken wings in a bowl and mix until well coated and set aside for 20 minutes.
3. Preheat the oven to 450°F.
4. Spray a baking tray with cooking spray.
5. Place marinated wings on a prepared baking tray and bake for 30 minutes.
6. Serve and enjoy.

**NUTRITION:**

Calories: 355; Fat: 23g; Protein: 33g; Carbohydrates: 0.5g.

# LEMON CHICKEN

PREPARATION TIME: 10 MINUTES  |  COOKING TIME: 45 MINUTES  |  SERVINGS: 8

**INGREDIENTS:**

8 chicken breasts, skinless and boneless

¼ cup fresh lemon juice

2 tablespoons green onion, chopped

1 tablespoon oregano leaves

3 ounces feta cheese, crumbled

¼ teaspoon pepper

**DIRECTIONS:**

1. Preheat the oven to 350°F.
2. Spray baking dish with cooking spray.
3. Place chicken breasts in prepared baking dish.
4. Drizzle with 2 tablespoons lemon juice and sprinkle with 1/2 tablespoon oregano and pepper.
5. Top with green onion and crumbled cheese.
6. Drizzle with remaining lemon juice and oregano.
7. Bake for 45 minutes.
8. Serve and enjoy.

**NUTRITION:**

Calories: 246; Fat: 10.8g; Protein: 34g; Carbohydrates: 1.2g.

# TASTY SHREDDED CHICKEN

PREPARATION TIME: 10 MINUTES  |  COOKING TIME: 25 MINUTES  |  SERVINGS: 6

## INGREDIENTS:

3 chicken breasts, boneless and skinless

¼ cup vinegar

13.5 ounces chunky salsa

¼ teaspoon onion powder

1 tablespoon ground cumin

1 ½ tablespoons chili powder

## DIRECTIONS:

1.  Add all ingredients into the instant pot and stir well.

2.  Seal pot with lid and cook on manual high pressure for 25 minutes.

3.  Once done, release the pressure using the quick-release method, then open the lid.

4.  Remove chicken from pot and shred using a fork.

5.  Serve and enjoy.

## NUTRITION:

Calories: 171; Fat: 6.3g; Protein: 23g; Carbohydrates: 5g.

# CHICKEN BACON SALAD

PREPARATION TIME: 10 MINUTES | COOKING TIME: 10 MINUTES | SERVINGS: 4

## INGREDIENTS:

2 chicken breasts, cooked and chopped

3 bacon slices, cooked and chopped

½ cup celery, diced

2 avocado, chopped

2 ½ tablespoons olive oil

3 tablespoons fresh lemon juice

½ teaspoon dried dill

1 tablespoon dried chives

½ teaspoon pepper

1 teaspoon salt

## DIRECTIONS:

1. Add all ingredients into the large bowl and toss well to combine.

2. Serve and enjoy.

## NUTRITION:

Calories: 441; Fat: 36g; Protein: 24g; Carbohydrates: 10g.

# FLAVORFUL HERB CHICKEN

PREPARATION TIME: 10 MINUTES  |  COOKING TIME: 15 MINUTES  |  SERVINGS: 5

## INGREDIENTS:

2 pounds chicken breast, skinless and boneless

½ cup Greek yogurt

¼ cup mayonnaise

1 ½ teaspoons herb seasoning

½ teaspoon onion powder

½ teaspoon garlic powder

¼ teaspoon salt

## DIRECTIONS:

1. Preheat the air-fryer to 380°F.
2. In a small bowl, mix together mayonnaise, herb seasoning, onion powder, garlic powder, and yogurt.
3. Coat chicken with mayo mixture.
4. Spray air-fryer basket with cooking spray.
5. Place chicken in an air-fryer basket and cook for 15 minutes. Turn halfway through.
6. Serve and enjoy.

## NUTRITION:

Calories: 272; Fat: 8g; Protein: 40g; Carbohydrates: 5g.

# CARIBBEAN-STYLE CHICKEN WINGS

PREPARATION TIME: 10 MINUTES  |  COOKING TIME: 50 MINUTES  |  SERVINGS: 2

## INGREDIENTS:

4 chicken wings, skinless

1 tablespoon coconut aminos

2 tablespoons rum

2 tablespoons butter

1 tablespoon onion powder

1 tablespoon garlic powder

½ teaspoon salt

¼ teaspoon freshly ground black pepper

½ teaspoon red pepper flakes

¼ teaspoon dried dill

2 tablespoons sesame seeds

## DIRECTIONS:

1. Pat dry the chicken wings. Toss the chicken wings with the remaining ingredients until well coated. Arrange the chicken wings on a parchment-lined baking sheet.

2. Bake in the preheated oven at 430°F for 45 minutes until golden brown.

3. Serve with your favorite sauce for dipping. Bon appétit!

## NUTRITION:

Calories: 225; Fat: 18.5g; Protein: 15.6g; Carbohydrates: 5.2g.

# MEAT RECIPES

## COFFEE BUTTER RUBBED TRI-TIP STEAK

PREPARATION TIME: 20 MINUTES  |  COOKING TIME: 15 MINUTES  |  SERVINGS: 2

**INGREDIENTS:**

2 Tri-tip steaks, preferably ½ pound

1 package of coffee blocks

½ tablespoon garlic powder

1 teaspoon black pepper, coarse ground

2 tablespoons olive oil

½ tablespoon sea salt

**DIRECTIONS:**

1. Pound the meat using a mallet until tenderize; let the meat sit for 20 minutes at room temperature.

2. Combine everything together (except the steaks) in a large-sized mixing bowl.

3. Rub the sides, top, and bottom of the meat steaks entirely with the mixture.

4. Over medium-high heat in a large skillet; heat the olive oil until hot.

5. Carefully add the coated steaks into the hot oil and cook for 5 minutes.

6. Flip and cook the other side until cooked through, for 5 more minutes.

7. Remove the meat from the pan and let sit for a minute in its own juices.

8. Cut into slices against the grain. Serve warm and enjoy.

**NUTRITION:**

Calories: 371; Fat: 35g; Protein: 22g; Carbohydrates: 0.5g.

# KETO RIB EYE STEAK

PREPARATION TIME: 5 MINUTES  |  COOKING TIME: 20 MINUTES  |  SERVINGS: 2

## INGREDIENTS:

½ pound grass-fed rib-eye steak, preferably 1" thick

1 teaspoon Adobo Seasoning

1 tablespoon extra-virgin olive oil

Pepper and sea salt to taste

## DIRECTIONS:

1. Add steak in a large-sized mixing bowl and drizzle both sides with a small amount of olive oil.

2. Dust the seasonings on both sides; rubbing the seasonings into the meat.

3. Let sit for a couple of minutes and heat up your grill in advance.

4. Once hot; place the steaks over the grill, and cook until both sides are cooked through, for 15 to 20 minutes, flipping occasionally.

## NUTRITION:

Calories: 257; Fat: 19g; Protein: 24g; Carbohydrates: 0.3g.

# SPICY BEEF MEATBALLS

PREPARATION TIME: 10 MINUTES  |  COOKING TIME: 10 MINUTES  |  SERVINGS: 3

## INGREDIENTS:

1 cup mozzarella or cheddar cheese; cut into cubes

1 pound minced ground beef

1 teaspoon olive oil

3 tablespoons parmesan cheese

1 teaspoon garlic powder

½ teaspoon each of pepper, and salt

## DIRECTIONS:

1. Thoroughly combine the ground beef with the entire dry ingredients; mix well.

2. Wrap the cheese cubes into the mince; forming 9 meatballs from the prepared mixture.

3. Pan-fry the formed meatballs until cooked through, covered (uncover and stirring frequently).

## NUTRITION:

Calories: 595; Fat: 44g; Protein: 49g; Carbohydrates: 2.8g.

# TURKEY AND RADISHES

PREPARATION TIME: 5 MINUTES  |  COOKING TIME: 12 MINUTES  |  SERVINGS: 4

## INGREDIENTS:

1 tablespoon olive oil

1 pound radishes, trimmed and quartered

1 pound cooked turkey, chopped

1 onion, small, chopped

½ cup beef broth

Pepper and salt to taste

## DIRECTIONS:

1.  Over medium high heat settings in a large saucepan, heat a tablespoon of olive oil.

2.  Once hot, add and sauté the onion for a couple of minutes and then add the radishes; continue to sauté for 5 more minutes.

3.  Add in the beef broth; give everything a good stir until evenly mixed. Cover the pan loosely and cook until the liquid is reduced and the radishes are fork-tender for 5 minutes.

4.  Add in the cooked turkey. Season with pepper and salt to taste, giving everything a good stir. Serve immediately and enjoy.

## NUTRITION:

Calories: 304; Fat: 16g; Protein: 31g; Carbohydrates: 6.5g.

# SPICY STEAK CURRY

PREPARATION TIME: 15 MINUTES  |  COOKING TIME: 40 MINUTES  |  SERVINGS: 6

## INGREDIENTS:

1 cup plain yogurt

½ teaspoon garlic paste

½ teaspoon ginger paste

½ teaspoon ground cloves

½ teaspoon ground cumin

2 teaspoons red pepper flakes

¼ teaspoon ground turmeric

Salt

2 pounds grass-fed round steak

¼ cup olive oil

1 medium yellow onion

1 ½ tablespoons lemon juice

¼ cup cilantro

## DIRECTIONS:

1. Mix yogurt, garlic paste, ginger paste, and spices. Add the steak pieces. Set aside.

2. Sauté the onion for 4-5 minutes. Add the steak pieces with the marinade and mix.

3. Simmer for 25 minutes. Stir in the lemon juice and simmer 10 minutes.

4. Garnish with cilantro and serve.

## NUTRITION:

Calories: 440; Fat: 19g; Protein: 48.3g; Carbohydrates: 5.5g.

# BEEF STEW

PREPARATION TIME: 15 MINUTES  |  COOKING TIME: 1 HOUR 40 MINUTES  |  SERVINGS: 4

## INGREDIENTS:

1 1/3 pounds grass-fed chuck roast

Salt

Ground black pepper

2 tablespoons butter

1 yellow onion

2 garlic cloves

1 cup beef broth

1 bay leaf

½ teaspoon dried thyme

½ teaspoon dried rosemary

1 carrot

4 ounces celery stalks

1 tablespoon lemon juice

## DIRECTIONS:

1.  Put salt and black pepper in beef cubes.
2.  Sear the beef cubes for 4-5 minutes. Add the onion and garlic, then adjust the heat to medium and cook for 4-5 minutes. Add the broth, bay leaf, and dried herbs and boil.
3.  Simmer for 45 minutes. Stir in the carrot and celery and simmer for 30-45 minutes.
4.  Stir in lemon juice, salt, and black pepper. Serve.

## NUTRITION:

Calories: 413; Fat: 16g; Protein: 52g; Carbohydrates: 5.9g.

# BEEF & CABBAGE STEW

PREPARATION TIME: 15 MINUTES  |  COOKING TIME: 2 HOURS 10 MINUTES  |  SERVINGS: 8

**INGREDIENTS:**

2 pounds grass-fed beef stew meat

1 1/3 cups hot chicken broth

2 yellow onions

2 bay leaves

1 teaspoon Greek seasoning

Salt

Ground black pepper

3 celery stalks

1 package cabbage

1 can sugar-free tomato sauce

1 can sugar-free whole plum tomatoes

**DIRECTIONS:**

1. Sear the beef for 4-5 minutes. Stir in the broth, onion, bay leaves, Greek seasoning, salt, and black pepper and boil. Adjust the heat to low and cook for 1¼ hours.

2. Stir in the celery and cabbage and cook for 30 minutes. Stir in the tomato sauce and chopped plum tomatoes and cook, uncovered for 15-20 minutes. Stir in the salt, discard bay leaves and serve.

**NUTRITION:**

Calories: 247; Fat: 16g; Protein: 36.5g; Carbohydrates: 7g.

# STEAK WITH BLUEBERRY SAUCE

PREPARATION TIME: 15 MINUTES | COOKING TIME: 20 MINUTES | SERVINGS: 4

## INGREDIENTS:

### For sauce:

2 tablespoons butter

2 tablespoons yellow onion

2 garlic cloves

1 teaspoon thyme

1 1/3 cups beef broth

2 tablespoons lemon juice

¾ cup blueberries

### For steak:

2 tablespoons butter

4 grass-fed flank steaks

Salt

Ground black pepper

## DIRECTIONS:

1. For the sauce: sauté the onion for 2-3 minutes.

2. Add the garlic and thyme and sauté for 1 minute. Stir in the broth and simmer for 10 minutes.

3. For the steak: put salt and black pepper. Cook steaks for 3-4 minutes per side.

4. Transfer and put aside. Add sauce in the skillet and stir. Stir in the lemon juice, blueberries, salt, and black pepper and cook for 1-2 minutes. Put blueberry sauce over the steaks. Serve.

## NUTRITION:

Calories: 467; Fat: 19.7g; Protein: 49.5g; Carbohydrates: 5.7g

# BEEF TACO BAKE

PREPARATION TIME: 15 MINUTES  |  COOKING TIME: 1 HOUR  |  SERVINGS: 6

## INGREDIENTS:

### For crust:

3 organic eggs

4 ounces cream cheese

½ teaspoon taco seasoning

1/3 cup heavy cream

8 ounces cheddar cheese

### For topping:

1 pound grass-fed ground beef

4 ounces green chilies

¼ cup sugar-free tomato sauce

3 teaspoons taco seasoning

8 ounces cheddar cheese

## DIRECTIONS:

1. Warm-up oven to 375°F.
2. For the crust: beat the eggs, and cream cheese, taco seasoning, and heavy cream.
3. Place cheddar cheese in the baking dish. Spread cream cheese mixture over cheese.
4. Bake for 25-30 minutes. Remove, then set aside for 5 minutes.
5. For topping: Cook the beef for 8-10 minutes.
6. Stir in the green chilies, tomato sauce, and taco seasoning and transfer.
7. Place the beef mixture over the crust and sprinkle with cheese. Bake for 18-20 minutes.
8. Remove, then slice and serve.

## NUTRITION:

Calories: 569; Fat: g; Protein: 38.7g; Carbohydrates: 4g.

# MEATBALLS IN CHEESE SAUCE

PREPARATION TIME: 20 MINUTES | COOKING TIME: 25 MINUTES | SERVINGS: 5

## INGREDIENTS:

**For meatballs:**

1 pound ground pork

1 organic egg

2 ounces Parmesan cheese

½ tablespoon dried basil

1 teaspoon garlic powder

½ teaspoon onion powder

Salt

Ground black pepper

3 tablespoons olive oil

**For sauce:**

1 can sugar-free tomatoes

2 tablespoons butter

7 ounces spinach

2 tablespoons parsley

5 ounces mozzarella cheese

Salt

Ground black pepper

## DIRECTIONS:

1. For meatballs: Mix all the ingredients for the meatballs, except oil in a large bowl. Make small-sized balls from the mixture.

2. Cook the meatballs for 3-5 minutes. Add the tomatoes. Simmer for 15 minutes.

3. Stir fry the spinach for 1-2 minutes in butter. Add salt and black pepper.

4. Remove, then put the cooked spinach, parsley, and mozzarella cheese into meatballs and stir.

5. Cook for 1-2 minutes. Remove and serve.

## NUTRITION:

Calories: 398; Fat: 24.8g; Protein: 38.6g; Carbohydrates: 6.6g.

# CHOCOLATE CHILI

PREPARATION TIME: 15 MINUTES | COOKING TIME: 2 HOURS AND 15 MINUTES | SERVINGS: 8

## INGREDIENTS:

2 tablespoons olive oil

1 small onion

1 green bell pepper

4 garlic cloves

1 jalapeño pepper

1 teaspoon dried thyme

2 tablespoons red chili powder

1 tablespoon ground cumin

2 pounds lean ground pork

2 cups fresh tomatoes

4 ounces sugar-free tomato paste

1 ½ tablespoons cacao powder

2 cups chicken broth

1 cup water

Salt

Ground black pepper

¼ cup cheddar cheese

## DIRECTIONS:

1.  Sauté the onion and bell pepper for 5-7 minutes.
2.  Add the garlic, jalapeño pepper, thyme, and spices and sauté for 1 minute.
3.  Add the pork and cook for 4-5 minutes. Stir in the tomatoes, tomato paste, and cacao powder and cook for 2 minutes.
4.  Add the broth and water, boil. Simmer, covered for 2 hours. Stir in the salt and black pepper. Remove, then top with cheddar cheese and serve.

## NUTRITION:

Calories: 326; Fat: 22.9g; Protein: 23.3g; Carbohydrates: 9.1g.

# PORK STEW

PREPARATION TIME: 15 MINUTES  |  COOKING TIME: 45 MINUTES  |  SERVINGS: 6

**INGREDIENTS:**

2 tablespoons olive oil

2 pounds pork tenderloin

1 tablespoon garlic

2 teaspoons paprika

¾ cup chicken broth

1 cup sugar-free tomato sauce

½ tablespoon Erythritol

1 teaspoon dried oregano

2 dried bay leaves

2 tablespoons lemon juice

Salt

Ground black pepper

**DIRECTIONS:**

1. Cook the pork for 3-4 minutes. Add the garlic and cook for 1 minute.

2. Stir in the remaining fixing and boil. Simmer, covered for 30-40 minutes

3. Remove, then discard the bay leaves. Serve.

**NUTRITION:**

Calories: 277; Fat: 10.4g; Protein: 41g; Carbohydrates: 3.6g.

# PORK & CHILIES STEW

PREPARATION TIME: 15 MINUTES | COOKING TIME: 2 HOURS AND 10 MINUTES | SERVINGS: 8

## INGREDIENTS:

3 tablespoons unsalted butter

2 ½ pounds boneless pork ribs

1 large yellow onion

4 garlic cloves

1 ½ cups chicken broth

2 cans sugar-free tomatoes

1 cup canned roasted poblano chilies

2 teaspoons dried oregano

1 teaspoon ground cumin

Salt

¼ cup cilantro

2 tablespoons lime juice

## DIRECTIONS:

1. Cook the pork, onions, and garlic for 5 minutes.

2. Add the broth, tomatoes, poblano chilies, oregano, cumin, and salt and boil.

3. Simmer, covered for 2 hours. Mix with the fresh cilantro and lime juice and remove it. Serve.

## NUTRITION:

Calories: 288; Fat: 13.6g; Protein: 39.6g; Carbohydrates: 8.8g.

# SEAFOOD AND FISH RECIPES

## HERBED SEA BASS

PREPARATION TIME: 15 MINUTES | COOKING TIME: 20 MINUTES | SERVINGS: 2

**INGREDIENTS:**

2 (1¼-pound) whole sea bass; gutted, gilled, scaled, and fins removed

Salt and ground black pepper, to taste

6 fresh bay leaves

2 fresh thyme sprigs

2 fresh parsley sprigs

2 fresh rosemary sprigs

2 tablespoons butter, melted

2 tablespoons fresh lemon juice

**DIRECTIONS:**

1. Season the cavity and outer side of each fish with salt and black pepper evenly.
2. With plastic wrap, cover each fish and refrigerate for 1 hour.
3. Preheat the oven to 450°F.
4. Lightly grease a baking dish.
5. Arrange 2 bay leaves in the bottom of the prepared baking dish.
6. Divide herb sprigs and remaining bay leaves inside the cavity of each fish.
7. Arrange both fish over bay leaves in baking dish and drizzle with butter.
8. Roast for about 15–20 minutes or until fish is cooked through.
9. Remove the baking dish from the oven and place the fish onto a platter.
10. Drizzle the fish with lemon juice and serve.

**NUTRITION:**

Calories: 192; Fat: 6g; Protein: 29g; Carbohydrates: 4.2g.

# SUPER SALMON PARCEL

PREPARATION TIME: 15 MINUTES  |  COOKING TIME: 20 MINUTES  |  SERVINGS: 6

**INGREDIENTS:**

6 (3-ounce) salmon fillets

Salt and freshly ground black pepper, to taste

1 yellow bell pepper, seeded and cubed

1 red bell pepper, seeded and cubed

4 plum tomatoes, cubed

1 small yellow onion, sliced thinly

½ cup fresh parsley, chopped

¼ cup olive oil

2 tablespoons fresh lemon juice

**DIRECTIONS:**

1. Preheat the oven to 400°F.

2. Arrange 6 pieces of foil onto a smooth surface. Place 1 salmon fillet onto each foil piece and sprinkle with salt and black pepper. In a bowl, add the bell peppers, tomato and onion and mix. Place veggie mixture over each fillet evenly and top with parsley. Drizzle with oil and lemon juice. Fold the foil around salmon mixture to seal it. Arrange the foil packets onto a large baking sheet in a single layer. Bake for about 20 minutes.

3. Serve hot.

**NUTRITION:**

Calories: 224; Fat: 14g; Protein: 18.2g; Carbohydrates: 8.2g.

# JUICY GARLIC BUTTER SHRIMP

PREPARATION TIME: 10 MINUTES  |  COOKING TIME: 5 MINUTES  |  SERVINGS: 4

## INGREDIENTS:

2 pounds shrimp, peeled and deveined

2 tablespoons fresh herbs, chopped

2 tablespoons fresh lemon juice

1 teaspoon paprika

1 tablespoon garlic, minced

¼ cup butter

Pepper

Salt

## DIRECTIONS:

1.  Melt butter in a pan over medium heat.

2.  Add garlic and sauté for 30 seconds.

3.  Add shrimp, paprika, pepper, and salt. Cook shrimp for 2 minutes on each side.

4.  Add remaining ingredients, stir well and cook for 1 minute.

5.  Serve and enjoy.

## NUTRITION:

Calories: 379; Fat: 15.5g; Protein: 52.1g; Carbohydrates: 5g.

# EASY BAKED SHRIMP SCAMPI

PREPARATION TIME: 10 MINUTES  |  COOKING TIME: 10 MINUTES  |  SERVINGS: 4

**INGREDIENTS:**

2 pounds shrimp, peeled

¾ cup olive oil

2 teaspoons dried oregano

1 tablespoon garlic, minced

½ cup fresh lemon juice

¼ cup butter, sliced

Pepper

Salt

**DIRECTIONS:**

1. Preheat the oven to 350°F. Add shrimp in a baking dish. In a bowl, whisk together lemon juice, oregano, garlic, oil, pepper, and salt and pour over shrimp. Add butter on top of shrimp.

2. Bake in preheated oven for 10 minutes or until shrimp cooked. Serve and enjoy.

**NUTRITION:**

Calories: 708; Fat: 53.5g; Protein: 52.2g; Carbohydrates: 5.3g.

# FLAVORFUL SHRIMP CREOLE

PREPARATION TIME: 10 MINUTES | COOKING TIME: 1 HOUR 30 MINUTES | SERVINGS: 8

## INGREDIENTS:

2 pounds shrimp, peeled

¾ cup green onions, chopped

1 teaspoon garlic, minced

2 ½ cups water

1 tablespoon hot sauce

8 ounces can tomato sauce, sugar-free

8 ounces can tomato paste

½ cup bell pepper, chopped

¾ cup celery, chopped

1 cup onion, chopped

2 tablespoons olive oil

Pepper

Salt

## DIRECTIONS:

1. Heat oil in a saucepan over medium heat.
2. Add celery, onion, bell pepper, pepper, and salt and sauté until onion is softened.
3. Add tomato paste and cook for 5 minutes.
4. Add hot sauce, tomato sauce, and water and cook for 1 hour.
5. Add garlic and shrimp and cook for 15 minutes.
6. Add green onions and cook for 2 minutes more.
7. Serve and enjoy.

## NUTRITION:

Calories: 208; Fat: 5.7g; Protein: 27.92g; Carbohydrates: 11.6g.

# DELICIOUS BLACKENED SHRIMP

PREPARATION TIME: 10 MINUTES  |  COOKING TIME: 5 MINUTES  |  SERVINGS: 4

## INGREDIENTS:

1 ½ pounds shrimp, peeled

1 tablespoon garlic, minced

1 tablespoon olive oil

1 teaspoon garlic powder

1 teaspoon dried oregano

1 teaspoon cumin

1 tablespoon paprika

1 tablespoon chili powder

Pepper

Salt

## DIRECTIONS:

1. In a mixing bowl, mix together garlic powder, oregano, cumin, paprika, chili powder, pepper, and salt.
2. Add shrimp and mix until well-coated. Set aside for 30 minutes.
3. Heat oil in a pan over medium-high heat.
4. Add shrimp and cook for 2 minutes. Turn shrimp and cook for 2 minutes more.
5. Add garlic and cook for 30 seconds.
6. Serve and enjoy.

## NUTRITION:

Calories: 252; Fat: 7.1g; Protein: 39.6g; Carbohydrates: 6.3g.

# SIMPLE LEMON GARLIC SHRIMP

PREPARATION TIME: 5 MINUTES  |  COOKING TIME: 15 MINUTES  |  SERVINGS: 4

## INGREDIENTS:

1 ½ pounds shrimp, peeled and deveined

¼ cup fresh parsley, chopped

¼ cup fresh lemon juice

1 tablespoon garlic, minced

¼ cup butter

Pepper

Salt

## DIRECTIONS:

1.  Melt butter in a pan over medium heat. Add garlic and sauté for 30 seconds.
2.  Add shrimp and season with pepper and salt and cook for 4-5 minutes or until it turns to pink.
3.  Add lemon juice and parsley, stir well and cook for 2 minutes. Serve and enjoy.

## NUTRITION:

Calories: 312; Fat: 14.6g; Protein: 39.2g; Carbohydrates: 3.9g.

# PERFECT PAN-SEARED SCALLOPS

PREPARATION TIME: 10 MINUTES  |  COOKING TIME: 4 MINUTES  |  SERVINGS: 4

**INGREDIENTS:**

1 pound scallops, rinse and pat dry

1 tablespoon olive oil

2 tablespoons butter

Pepper

Salt

**DIRECTIONS:**

1. Season scallops with pepper and salt.

2. Heat butter and oil in a pan over medium heat.

3. Add scallops and sear for 2 minutes, then turn to other side and cook for 2 minutes more.

4. Serve and enjoy.

**NUTRITION:**

Calories: 181; Fat: 10.1g; Protein: 19.1g; Carbohydrates: 2.7g.

# SALAD RECIPES

# BACON AVOCADO SALAD

PREPARATION TIME: 20 MINUTES  |  COOKING TIME: 0 MINUTES  |  SERVINGS: 4

## INGREDIENTS:

2 hard-boiled eggs, chopped

2 cups spinach

2 large avocados, 1 chopped and 1 sliced

2 small lettuce heads, chopped

1 spring onion, sliced

4 cooked bacon slices, crumbled

**For the vinaigrette:**

Olive oil

Mustard

Apple cider vinegar

## DIRECTIONS:

1. In a large bowl, mix the eggs, spinach, avocados, lettuce, and onion. Set aside.
2. Make the vinaigrette: In a separate bowl, add the olive oil, mustard, and apple cider vinegar. Mix well.
3. Pour the vinaigrette into the large bowl and toss well.
4. Serve topped with bacon slices and sliced avocado.

## NUTRITION:

Calories: 268; Fat: 16.9g; Protein: 5g; Carbohydrates: 8g.

# CAULIFLOWER, SHRIMP, AND CUCUMBER SALAD

PREPARATION TIME: 10 MINUTES | COOKING TIME: 15 MINUTES | SERVINGS: 6

## INGREDIENTS:

¼ cup olive oil

1 pound (454 g) medium shrimp

1 cauliflower head, florets only

2 cucumbers, peeled and chopped

**For the dressing:**

Olive oil

Lemon juice

Lemon zest

Dill

Salt and pepper

## DIRECTIONS:

1. In a skillet over medium heat, heat the olive oil until sizzling hot. Add the shrimp and cook for 8 minutes, stirring occasionally, or until the flesh is pink and opaque.

2. Meanwhile, in a microwave-safe bowl, add the cauliflower florets and microwave for about 5 minutes until tender.

3. Remove the shrimp from the heat to a large bowl. Add the cauliflower and cucumber to the shrimp in the bowl. Set aside.

4. Make the dressing: Mix the olive oil, lemon juice, lemon zest, dill, salt, and pepper in a third bowl. Pour the dressing into the bowl of shrimp mixture. Toss well until the shrimp and vegetables are coated thoroughly.

5. Serve immediately or refrigerate for 1 hour before serving.

## NUTRITION:

Calories: 308; Fat: 19g; Protein: 5g; Carbohydrates: 4g.

# BACON BLEU ZOODLE SALAD

PREPARATION TIME: 5 MINUTES  |  COOKING TIME: 0 MINUTES  |  SERVINGS: 2

**INGREDIENTS:**

4 cups zucchini noodles

½ cup bacon, cooked and crumbled

1 cup fresh spinach, chopped

1/3 cup bleu cheese, crumbled

Fresh cracked pepper, to taste

**DIRECTIONS:**

1. Toss the entire ingredients together in a large-sized mixing bowl. Serve immediately, and enjoy.

**NUTRITION:**

Calories: 214; Fat: 17g; Protein: 33g; Carbohydrates: 6g.

# SALMON AND LETTUCE SALAD

PREPARATION TIME: 10 MINUTES | COOKING TIME: 0 MINUTES | SERVINGS: 4

**INGREDIENTS:**

1 tablespoon extra-virgin olive oil

2 salmon fillets, chopped

3 tablespoons mayonnaise

1 tablespoon lime juice

Sea salt, to taste

1 cup romaine lettuce, shredded

1 teaspoon onion flakes

½ avocado, sliced

**DIRECTIONS:**

1. In a bowl, stir together the olive oil, salmon, mayo, lime juice, and salt. Stir well until the salmon is coated fully.

2. Divide evenly the romaine lettuce and onion flakes among four serving plates. Spread the salmon mixture over the lettuce, then serve topped with avocado slices.

**NUTRITION:**

Calories: 271; Fat: 18g; Protein: 6g; Carbohydrates: 4g.

# SHRIMP, TOMATO, AND AVOCADO SALAD

PREPARATION TIME: 5 MINUTES  |  COOKING TIME: 0 MINUTES  |  SERVINGS: 4

## INGREDIENTS:

1 pound (454 g) shrimp, shelled and deveined

2 tomatoes, cubed

2 avocados, peeled and cubed

A handful of fresh cilantro, chopped

4 green onions, minced

Juice of 1 lime or lemon

1 tablespoon macadamia nut or avocado oil

Celtic sea salt and fresh ground black pepper, to taste

## DIRECTIONS:

1. Combine the shrimp, tomatoes, avocados, cilantro, and onions in a large bowl.
2. Squeeze the lemon juice over the vegetables in the large bowl, then drizzle with avocado oil and sprinkle the salt and black pepper to season. Toss to combine well.
3. You can cover the salad, and refrigerate to chill for 45 minutes or serve immediately.

## NUTRITION:

Calories: 158; Fat: 10g; Protein: 9g; Carbohydrates: 4g.

# CHILI-LIME TUNA SALAD

PREPARATION TIME: 10 MINUTES  |  COOKING TIME: 0 MINUTES  |  SERVINGS: 2

## INGREDIENTS:

1 tablespoon lime juice

1/3 cup mayonnaise

¼ teaspoon salt

1 teaspoon Tajin chili lime seasoning

1/8 teaspoon pepper

1 medium stalk celery (finely chopped)

2 cups romaine lettuce (chopped roughly)

2 tablespoons red onion (finely chopped)

Optional: chopped green onion, black pepper, lemon juice

5 ounces canned tuna

## DIRECTIONS:

1. Using a bowl of medium size, mix some of the ingredients, such as lime, pepper, and chili-lime.

2. Then, add tuna and vegetables to the pot and stir. Enjoy!

## NUTRITION:

Calories: 259; Fat: 11.3g; Protein: 12.9g; Carbohydrates: 2.9g.

# PESTO CHICKEN SALAD

PREPARATION TIME: 4 MINUTES | COOKING TIME: 20 MINUTES | SERVINGS: 4

**INGREDIENTS:**

4 pieces chicken breast

½ cup of pesto

1 cup cherry tomatoes

3 cups spinach

A dash of salt

3 tablespoons olive oil

**DIRECTIONS:**

1. For another alternative for plain old, baked chicken, you will want to consider this delicious Pesto chicken salad! To start, prep the stove to 350°F. As this warms up, place your chicken pieces onto a baking plate and coat with the pepper, salt, and olive oil. When this is done, pop the dish into the oven for 40 minutes.

2. When the chicken is cooked through and no longer pink on the inside, take it out of the oven and cool slightly before handling.

3. Once you can handle the chicken, toss it into a bowl along with the pesto and your sliced tomatoes. When the ingredients are mixed to your liking, place over a bowl of fresh spinach and enjoy your salad.

**NUTRITION:**

Calories: 188; Fat: 19g; Protein: 20g; Carbohydrates: 5g.

# VEGETABLE RECIPES

## CAULIFLOWER RICE

PREPARATION TIME: 20 MINUTES  |  COOKING TIME: 8 MINUTES  |  SERVINGS: 2

**INGREDIENTS:**

1 head of cauliflower

1 tablespoon of olive oil or grass-fed butter

Salt to taste

**DIRECTIONS:**

1. Slice the cauliflower into small pieces with a sharp knife, add in a food processor, and process it until fully broken.
2. If any pieces are left unprocessed, put them back in and process them again.
3. Preheat a large pan and heat olive oil in it.
4. Add in your processed cauliflower with a pinch of salt.
5. Cover and cook for 4-8 minutes.
6. Then, serve warm.

**NUTRITION:**

Calories: 204; Fat: 11g; Protein: 1.5g; Carbohydrates: 4.2g.

# ROASTED OKRA

PREPARATION TIME: 3 MINUTES  |  COOKING TIME: 6 MINUTES  |  SERVINGS: 4

**INGREDIENTS:**

½ pound sliced okra

1 teaspoon olive oil

Salt and black pepper, to taste

**DIRECTIONS:**

1. Preheat the air fryer at 350°F for 5 min.
2. Season okra with olive oil, pepper, and salt.
3. Air fry for minutes, toss, and again air fry for 3 minutes. Relish.

**NUTRITION:**

Calories: 112; Fat: 5g; Protein: 4.7g; Carbohydrates:16g.

# PARMESAN ZUCCHINI FRIES

PREPARATION TIME: 5 MINUTES  |  COOKING TIME: 20 MINUTES  |  SERVINGS: 2

**INGREDIENTS:**

1 thinly sliced Zucchini

1 large beaten egg

¾ cup crated Parmesan cheese

1 cup panko bread crumbs

**DIRECTIONS:**

1. First, preheat the air fryer at 350°F.
2. Mix panko bread crumbs and parmesan cheese. Dip zucchini in egg and then coat with panko bread crumbs mixture. Gently press to firm the coating.
3. Air fry the zucchini fries for 10 minutes, shake the air fryer basket, and again air fry for 5 minutes.
4. Serve with coleslaw. Relish.

**NUTRITION:**

Calories: 160; Fat: 6.5g; Protein: 10.9g; Carbohydrates: 21g.

# CREAMY ZOODLES

PREPARATION TIME: 15 MINUTES  |  COOKING TIME: 10 MINUTES  |  SERVINGS: 4

## INGREDIENTS:

1 cup heavy whipping cream

1/4 cup mayonnaise

Salt and ground black pepper, as required

30 ounces zucchini, spiralized with blade C

3 ounces Parmesan cheese, grated

2 tablespoons fresh mint leaves

2 tablespoons butter, melted

## DIRECTIONS:

1. The heavy cream must be added to a pan then bring to a boil.
2. Lower the heat to low and cook until reduced in half.
3. Put in the pepper, mayo, and salt; cook until the mixture is warm enough.
4. Add the zucchini noodles and gently stir to combine.
5. Stir in the Parmesan cheese.
6. Divide the zucchini noodles onto four serving plates and immediately drizzle with the melted butter.
7. Serve immediately.

## NUTRITION:

Calories: 241; Fat: 11.4g; Protein: 5.1g; Carbohydrates: 3.1g.

# BAKED ZUCCHINI GRATIN

PREPARATION TIME: 25 MINUTES  |  COOKING TIME: 25 MINUTES  |  SERVINGS: 2

## INGREDIENTS:

1 large zucchini, cut into 1/4-inch-thick slices

1 ounce Brie cheese, rind trimmed off

1 tablespoon butter

Freshly ground black pepper

1/3 cup shredded Gruyere cheese

1/4 cup crushed pork rinds

## DIRECTIONS:

1. Preheat the oven to 400°F.
2. When the zucchini has been "weeping" for about 30 minutes, in a small saucepan over medium-low heat, heat the Brie and butter, occasionally stirring, until the cheese has melted.
3. The mixture is thoroughly combined for about 2 minutes.
4. Arrange the zucchini in an 8-inch baking dish, so the zucchini slices are overlapping a bit.
5. Season with pepper.
6. Pour the Brie mixture over the zucchini, and top with the shredded Gruyere cheese.
7. Sprinkle the crushed pork rinds over the top.
8. Bake for about 25 minutes, until the dish is bubbling and the top is nicely browned, and serve.

## NUTRITION:

Calories: 324; Fat: 11.5g; Protein: 5.1g; Carbohydrates: 2.2g.

# AVOCADO CHIPS

PREPARATION TIME: 4 MINUTES  |  COOKING TIME: 8 MINUTES  |  SERVINGS: 2

## INGREDIENTS:

1 de-seeded, peeled, sliced avocado

½ cup panko bread crumbs

¼ cup coconut flour

1 large beaten egg

1 teaspoon water

¼ teaspoon kosher salt

Cooking spray

## DIRECTIONS:

1. First, preheat the air fryer to 400°F. Spray basket with cooking spray

2. Combine flour and salt in a container, egg and water in another, and panko bread crumbs in the last container. Dredge avocado slices in each, respectively.

3. Air fry for 4 minutes, flip the sides, and again fry until golden brown.

## NUTRITION:

Calories: 320; Fat: 18g; Protein: 9.2g; Carbohydrates: 40g.

# BAKED RADISHES

PREPARATION TIME: 10 MINUTES  |  COOKING TIME: 20 MINUTES  |  SERVINGS: 4

## INGREDIENTS:

1 tablespoon chopped chives

15 sliced radishes

Salt

Vegetable oil cooking spray

Black pepper

## DIRECTIONS:

1. Line your baking sheet well, then spray with the cooking spray.

2. Set the sliced radishes on the baking tray then sprinkle with cooking oil.

3. Add the seasonings then top with chives.

4. Set the oven for 10 minutes at 375°F, allow to bake.

5. Turn the radishes to bake for 10 minutes. Serve cold.

## NUTRITION:

Calories: 63; Fat: 8g; Protein: 1g; Carbohydrates: 6g.

# RELATIVELY FLAVORED GRATIN

PREPARATION TIME: 15 MINUTES  |  COOKING TIME: 46 MINUTES  |  SERVINGS: 8

**INGREDIENTS:**

½ cup heavy whipping cream

2 tablespoons butter

½ teaspoon garlic powder

¼ teaspoon xanthan gum

4 cups zucchini, sliced

1 small yellow onion, thinly sliced

Salt and freshly ground black pepper, to taste

1 ½ cups pepper jack cheese, shredded

**DIRECTIONS:**

1. Preheat the oven to 375°F and grease a 9×9-inch baking dish.
2. In a microwave-safe dish, place the heavy whipping cream, butter, garlic powder, and xanthan gum and microwave for about 1 minute.
3. Remove from microwave and beat the mixture until smooth.
4. Arrange 1/3 of zucchini and onion slices in the bottom of prepared baking dish and sprinkle with some salt, black pepper and cup pepper jack cheese.
5. Repeat the layers twice.
6. Now, place the cream mixture evenly on top.
7. Bake for about 45 minutes or until the top is golden brown.
8. Remove the baking dish from oven and set aside for about 5-10 minutes before serving.
9. Cut into 8 equal-sized portions and serve.

**NUTRITION:**

Calories: 140; Fat: 11.8g; Protein: 5.5g; Carbohydrates: 3.9g.

# THANKSGIVING VEGGIE MEAL

PREPARATION TIME: 20 MINUTES | COOKING TIME: 30 MINUTES | SERVINGS: 6

## INGREDIENTS:

**For onion slices:**

½ cup yellow onion, sliced very thinly

¼ cup almond flour

1/8 teaspoon garlic powder

Salt and freshly ground black pepper, to taste

**For casserole:**

1 pound fresh green beans, trimmed

1 tablespoon olive oil

8 ounces. fresh cremini mushrooms, sliced

½ cup yellow onion, thinly sliced

1/8 teaspoon garlic powder

Salt and freshly ground black pepper, to taste

1 teaspoon fresh thyme, chopped

½ cup homemade vegetable broth

½ cup sour cream

## DIRECTIONS:

1. Preheat the oven to 350°F.
2. For onion slices: in a bowl, place all the ingredients and toss to coat well.
3. Arrange the onion slices onto a large baking sheet in a single layer.
4. In a pan of salted boiling water, add the green beans and cook for about 5 minutes.
5. Drain the green beans and transfer into a bowl of ice water.
6. Again, drain well and transfer into a large bowl.
7. In a large skillet, heat the oil over medium-high heat and sauté the mushrooms, onion, garlic powder, salt and black pepper for about 2-3 minutes.
8. Stir in the thyme, and broth and cook for about 3-5 minutes or until all the liquid is absorbed.
9. Remove from heat and transfer the mushroom mixture into the bowl with green beans.
10. Add the sour cream and stir to combine well.
11. Transfer the mixture into a 10-inch casserole dish.
12. Place the casserole dish and baking sheet of onion slices into the oven.
13. Bake for about 15-17 minutes.
14. Remove the baking dish from oven and let it cool for about 5 minutes before serving.
15. Top the casserole evenly with crispy onion slices.
16. Cut into 6 equal-sized portions and serve.

## NUTRITION:

Calories: 134; Fat: 8.8g; Protein: 4.6g; Carbohydrates: 10g.

# SOUP AND STEW RECIPES

## IDEAL COLD WEATHER STEW

COOKING TIME: 2 HOURS 40 MINUTES | PREPARATION TIME: 20 MINUTES | SERVINGS: 6

**INGREDIENTS:**

3 tablespoons olive oil, divided

8 ounces fresh mushrooms, quartered

1 ¼ pounds grass-fed beef chuck roast, trimmed and cubed into 1-inch size

2 tablespoons tomato paste

½ teaspoon dried thyme

1 bay leaf

5 cups homemade beef broth

6 ounces celery root, peeled and cubed

4 ounces yellow onions, chopped roughly

3 ounces carrot, peeled and sliced

2 garlic cloves, sliced

Salt and freshly ground black pepper, to taste

**DIRECTIONS:**

1. In a Dutch oven, heat 1 tablespoons of oil over medium heat and cook the mushrooms for about 2 minutes without stirring.

2. Stir the mushroom and cook for about 2 minutes more.

3. With a slotted spoon, transfer the mushroom onto a plate.

4. In the same pan, heat the remaining oil over medium-high heat and sear the beef cubes for about 4-5 minutes.

5. Stir in the tomato paste, thyme, and bay leaf and cook for about 1 minute.

6. Stir in the broth and bring to a boil.

7. Reduce the heat to low and simmer, covered for about 1½ hours.

8. Stir in the mushrooms, celery, onion, carrot, and garlic and simmers for about 40-60 minutes.

9. Stir in the salt and black pepper and remove from the heat.

10. Serve hot.

**NUTRITION:**

Calories: 447; Fat: 7.4g; Protein: 30.8g; Carbohydrates: 7.4g.

# HUNGARIAN PORK STEW

COOKING TIME: 2 HOURS 20 MINUTES  |  PREPARATION TIME: 15 MINUTES  |  SERVINGS: 10

## INGREDIENTS:

3 tablespoons olive oil

3 ½ pounds pork shoulder, cut into 4 portions

1 tablespoon butter

2 medium onions, chopped

16 ounces tomatoes, crushed

5 garlic cloves, crushed

2 Hungarian wax peppers, chopped

3 tablespoons Hungarian Sweet paprika

1 tablespoon smoked paprika

1 teaspoon hot paprika

½ teaspoon caraway seeds

1 bay leaf

1 cup homemade chicken broth

1 packet unflavored gelatin

2 tablespoons fresh lemon juice

Pinch of xanthan gum

Salt and freshly ground black pepper, to taste

## DIRECTIONS:

1. In a heavy-bottomed pan, heat 1 tablespoon of oil over high heat and sear the pork for about 2-3 minutes or until browned.
2. Transfer the pork onto a plate and cut it into bite-sized pieces.
3. In the same pan, heat 1 tablespoon of oil and butter over medium-low heat and sauté the onions for about 5-6 minutes.
4. With a slotted spoon, transfer the onion into a bowl.
5. In the same pan, add the tomatoes and cook for about 3-4 minutes, without stirring.
6. Meanwhile, in a small frying pan, heat the remaining oil over low heat and sauté the garlic, wax peppers, all kinds of paprika, and caraway seeds for about 20-30 seconds.
7. Remove from the heat and set aside.
8. In a small bowl, mix together the gelatin and broth.
9. In the large pan, add the cooked pork, garlic mixture, gelatin mixture, and bay leaf and bring to a gentle boil.
10. Reduce the heat to low and simmer, covered for about 2 hours.
11. Stir in the xanthan gum and simmer for about 3-5 minutes.
12. Stir in the lemon juice, salt, and black pepper and remove from the heat.
13. Serve hot.

## NUTRITION:

Calories: 529; Fat: 38.5g; Protein: 38.9g; Carbohydrates: 5.8g.

# WILD MUSHROOM SOUP

PREPARATION TIME: 10 MINUTES  |  COOKING TIME: 30 MINUTES  |  SERVINGS: 4

**INGREDIENTS:**

6 ounces mix of portabella mushrooms, oyster mushrooms, and shiitake mushrooms

3 cups water

1 garlic clove

1 shallot

4 ounces butter

1 chicken bouillon cube

½ pound celery root

1 teaspoon thyme

1 tablespoon white wine vinegar

1 cup heavy whipping cream

Fresh parsley

**DIRECTIONS:**

1. Clean, trim, and chop your mushrooms and celery. Do the same to your shallot and garlic.
2. Sauté your chopped veggies in butter over medium heat in a saucepan.
3. Add thyme, vinegar, chicken bouillon cube, and water as you bring to boil. Then let it simmer for 10-15 minutes.
4. Add cream to them with an immersion blender until your desired consistency. Serve with parsley on top.

**NUTRITION:**

Calories: 481; Fat: 47g; Protein: 7g; Carbohydrates: 9g.

# ZUCCHINI CREAM SOUP

PREPARATION TIME: 5 MINUTES  |  COOKING TIME: 20 MINUTES  |  SERVINGS: 4

**INGREDIENTS:**

3 zucchinis

32 ounces chicken broth

2 cloves garlic

2 tablespoons sour cream

½ small onion

Parmesan cheese (for topping if desired)

**DIRECTIONS:**

1. Combine your broth, garlic, zucchini, and onion in a large pot over medium heat until boiling.

2. Lower the heat, cover, and let simmer for 15-20 minutes.

3. Remove from heat and purée with an immersion blender, while adding the sour cream and pureeing until smooth.

4. Season to taste and top with your cheese.

**NUTRITION:**

Calories: 117; Fat: 9g; Protein: 4g; Carbohydrates: 3g.

# CAULIFLOWER SOUP

PREPARATION TIME: 5 MINUTES  |  COOKING TIME: 25 MINUTES  |  SERVINGS: 6

## INGREDIENTS:

32 ounces vegetable broth

1 head cauliflower, diced

2 garlic cloves, minced

1 onion, diced

½ tablespoon olive oil

Salt and pepper

Grated Parmesan, sliced green onion for topping

## DIRECTIONS:

1. In a pot, heat oil over medium heat, while adding the onion and garlic. Then cook them for 4-5 minutes.

2. Add in the cauliflower and vegetable broth. Boil it and then cover for 15-20 minutes while covered.

3. Pour all contents of pot into a blender and season it.

4. Blend until smooth. Top it with your cheese and green onion.

## NUTRITION:

Calories: 37; Fat: 1g; Protein: 3g; Carbohydrates: 3g.

# THAI COCONUT SOUP

PREPARATION TIME: 10 MINUTES  |  COOKING TIME: 35 MINUTES  |  SERVINGS: 4

## INGREDIENTS:

3 chicken breasts

9 ounces coconut milk

9 ounces chicken broth

2/3 tablespoon chili sauce

18 ounces water

2/3 tablespoon coconut aminos

2/3 ounce lime juice

2/3 teaspoon ground ginger

¼ cup red boat fish sauce

Salt and pepper

## DIRECTIONS:

1. Slice up the chicken breasts thinly. Make them bite-sized.

2. In a large stock pot, mix your coconut milk, water, fish sauce, chili sauce, lime juice, ginger, coconut aminos, and broth. Bring to a boil.

3. Stir in chicken pieces. Then reduce the heat and cover pot, while simmering for 30 minutes.

4. Season them and enjoy.

## NUTRITION:

Calories: 227; Fat: 17g; Protein: 19g; Carbohydrates: 3g.

# CHICKEN RAMEN SOUP

PREPARATION TIME: 10 MINUTES  |  COOKING TIME: 20 MINUTES  |  SERVINGS: 2

**INGREDIENTS:**

1 chicken breast

2 eggs

1 zucchini, made into noodles

4 cups chicken broth

2 cloves garlic, peeled and minced

2 tablespoons coconut aminos

3 tablespoons avocado oil

1 tablespoon ginger

**DIRECTIONS:**

1. Pan-fry the chicken in avocado oil in a pan until brown.

2. Hard boil your eggs and slice them in half.

3. Add chicken broth to a large pot and simmer with the garlic, coconut aminos, and ginger. Then add in the zucchini noodles for 4-5 minutes.

4. Put the broth into a bowl, top it with eggs and chicken slices, and season to your liking.

**NUTRITION:**

Calories: 478; Fat: 39g; Protein: 31g; Carbohydrates: 3g.

# CREAMY MIXED SEAFOOD SOUP

PREPARATION TIME: 15 MINUTES  |  COOKING TIME: 15 MINUTES  |  SERVINGS: 4

## INGREDIENTS:

1 tablespoon avocado oil

2 garlic cloves, minced

¾ tablespoon almond flour

1 cup vegetable broth

1 teaspoon dried dill

1 pound frozen mixed seafood

Salt and black pepper to taste

1 tablespoon plain vinegar

2 cups cooking cream

Fresh dill leaves to garnish

## DIRECTIONS:

1. Heat oil, sauté the garlic for 30 seconds or until fragrant.
2. Stir in the almond flour until brown.
3. Mix in the vegetable broth until smooth and stir in the dill, seafood mix, salt, and black pepper.
4. Bring the soup to a boil and then simmer for 3 to 4 minutes or until the seafood cooks.
5. Add the vinegar, cooking cream, and stir well. Garnish with dill, serve.

## NUTRITION:

Calories: 361; Fat: 12.4g; Protein: 11.7g; Carbohydrates: 3.9g.

# DESSERT RECIPES

## COCONUT PUDDING

PREPARATION TIME: 15 MINUTES | COOKING TIME: 5 MINUTES | SERVINGS: 4

### INGREDIENTS:

1 ½ cups unsweetened almond milk, divided

1 tablespoon unflavored powdered gelatin

1 cup unsweetened coconut milk

1/3 cup Swerve

3 tablespoons cacao powder

2 teaspoons instant coffee granules

6 drops liquid stevia

### DIRECTIONS:

1. In a large bowl, add 1/2 cup of almond milk and sprinkle evenly with gelatin.
2. Set aside until soaked.
3. In a pan, add the remaining almond milk, coconut milk, Swerve, cacao powder, coffee granules, and stevia and bring to a gentle boil, stirring continuously.
4. Remove from the heat.
5. In a blender, add the gelatin mixture, and hot milk mixture and pulse until smooth.
6. Transfer the mixture into serving glasses and set aside to cool completely.
7. With plastic wrap, cover each glass and refrigerate for about 3-4 hours before serving.

### NUTRITION:

Calories: 136; Fat: 12.1g; Protein: 4.4g; Carbohydrates: 5.8g.

# PRETTY BLUEBERRY BITES

PREPARATION TIME: 20 MINUTES  |  COOKING TIME: 0 MINUTES  |  SERVINGS: 10

## INGREDIENTS:

1 scoop unsweetened whey Protein powder

½ cup coconut flour, sifted

1-2 tablespoon granulated Erythritol

¼ teaspoon ground cinnamon

Pinch of salt

¼ cup dried unsweetened blueberries

½-1 cup unsweetened almond milk

## DIRECTIONS:

1. Line a large baking sheet with parchment paper. Set aside.
2. In a large bowl, add the protein powder, flour, Erythritol, cinnamon, and salt and mix well.
3. Add the blueberries and stir to combine.
4. Gradually, add the desired amount of the almond milk and mix until a dough is formed.
5. Immediately, make desired sized balls from the blueberry mixture.
6. Arrange the balls onto the prepared baking sheet in a single layer.
7. Refrigerate to set for about 30 minutes before serving.

## NUTRITION:

Calories: 18; Fat: 0.4g; Protein: 2.4g; Carbohydrates: 1.3g.

# COLD MINI MUFFINS

PREPARATION TIME: 20 MINUTES | COOKING TIME: 2 MINUTES | SERVINGS: 24

**INGREDIENTS:**

20 ounces 70% dark chocolate chips, divided

¼ cup coconut butter, softened

24 whole almonds

**DIRECTIONS:**

1. Line 24 cups of a mini muffin tin with paper liners. Set aside.
2. In a microwave-safe bowl, add 3/4 of chocolate chips and microwave on High for about 1 minute, stirring once halfway through.
3. Remove from microwave and stir well.
4. Divide the melted chocolate into prepared muffin cups evenly and refrigerate until set completely.
5. In a microwave-safe bowl, add the remaining chocolate chips and microwave on High for about 1 minute, stirring once halfway through.
6. Remove from microwave and stir well.
7. Remove from the refrigerator and t top each chocolate cup with the softened coconut butter evenly, followed by the remaining melted chocolate.
8. Gently, insert 1 almond in each cup and refrigerate until set before serving.

**NUTRITION:**

Calories: 151; Fat: 14.7g; Protein: 3.6g; Carbohydrates: 7.1g.

# CHOCOLATE LOVER'S MUFFINS

PREPARATION TIME: 15 MINUTES  |  COOKING TIME: 20 MINUTES  |  SERVINGS: 6

**INGREDIENTS:**

4 tablespoons almond flour

2 tablespoons coconut flour

2 tablespoons beet powder

1 tablespoon organic baking powder

2 organic eggs

1 teaspoon liquid stevia

3 tablespoons unsweetened almond milk

1/2 teaspoon organic vanilla extract

1/3 cup 70% dark chocolate

**DIRECTIONS:**

1. Preheat the oven to 375°F. Grease 6 cups of a muffin tin.
2. In a bowl, add the flours, beet powder and baking powder and mix well.
3. In another large bowl, add the eggs, stevia, almond milk and vanilla extract and beat until well-combined.
4. Add the flour mixture and mix until just combined.
5. Gently, fold in the chocolate chips.
6. Place the mixture into the prepared muffin cups evenly.
7. Bake for about 15-20 minutes or until a toothpick inserted in the center comes out clean.
8. Remove from the oven and place the muffin tin onto a wire rack to cool for about 10 minutes.
9. Carefully invert the muffins onto the wire rack to cool completely before serving.

**NUTRITION:**

Calories: 152; Fat: 9.9g; Protein: 5.2g; Carbohydrates: 10.2g.

# COCOA BROWNIES

PREPARATION TIME: 10 MINUTES | COOKING TIME: 30 MINUTES | SERVINGS: 9 SERVINGS

**INGREDIENTS:**

½ cup salted butter, melted

1 cup Granular Swerve Sweetener

2 large eggs

2 teaspoons vanilla extract

12 squares unsweetened baking chocolate, melted

2 tablespoons coconut flour

2 tablespoons cocoa powder

½ teaspoon baking powder

½ teaspoon salt

½ cup walnuts, chopped (optional)

**DIRECTIONS:**

1. Preheat oven to 350°F.
2. Spray square baking pan with cooking spray or grease pan well with butter.
3. In a large mixing bowl, use an electric mixer or whisk and mix together butter and sweetener.
4. Add the eggs and vanilla extract to bowl and mix with an electric mixer for 1 minute until smooth.
5. Add melted chocolate and stir with a wooden spoon or spatula until the chocolate is incorporated into the butter mixture.
6. In a separate bowl, mix the dry ingredients (remaining ingredients besides walnuts) until combined.
7. Add dry ingredients into the bowl with the wet ingredients and stir with a wooden spoon until combined.
8. Add walnuts if desired.
9. Pour batter into prepared pan. Spread to cover the entire bottom of the pan and into corners.
10. Place in the center rack of the oven and bake for 30 minutes.
11. After the brownies are baked, take them out and leave them in the pan to cool.
12. When cool, cut them into 9 servings, and they are ready to eat.
13. These have to be as a once-in-a-while treat because they are sweet, and if you're like me, that sugar will continue to call your name. These are so good you will have to work to eat only one serving.

**NUTRITION:**

Calories: 201; Fat: 19g; Protein: 3g; Carbohydrates: 5g.

# CHOCOLATE CHIP COOKIES

PREPARATION TIME: 10 MINUTES  |  COOKING TIME: 20 MINUTES  |  SERVINGS: 24 COOKIES

## INGREDIENTS:

1 ½ cups almond flour

1 teaspoon baking powder

½ teaspoon salt

½ cup butter, softened

½ cup stevia

1 teaspoon vanilla extract

1 large egg

1 cup sugar-free chocolate chips

½ cup nuts, chopped

## DIRECTIONS:

1.  Preheat oven to 350°F.

2.  Grease cookie sheets with butter and set aside.

3.  In a large bowl, cream together the butter and the stevia.

4.  Add the large egg and vanilla extract to the butter and stevia.

5.  Mix until the egg is incorporated into the butter.

6.  In a second bowl, mix together almond flour, baking powder, and salt until mixed well.

7.  Add dry ingredients to the large bowl and mix until it is combined.

8.  Add sugar-free chocolate chips and nuts and stir until they are distributed evenly.

9.  Drop by spoonfuls onto the cookie sheet.

10. Bake until golden brown and the surface of cookies appear dry on the top and are cooked all the way through.

11. Remove cookies from sheet to a wire rack to cool.

12. Make these with or without nuts. Cocoa nibs can be used in place of the sugar-free chocolate chips. This is a good recipe to keep on hand, so you can have a cookie along with everyone else. Make it a fun project with kids or friends. Baking is always a good way to bring people together, and this is a recipe everyone will enjoy.

## NUTRITION:

Calories: 120; Fat: 11g; Protein: 2g; Carbohydrates: 3g.

# KETO BROWN BUTTER PRALINES

PREPARATION TIME: 6 MINUTES  |  COOKING TIME: 10 MINUTES  |  SERVINGS: 10 SERVINGS

## INGREDIENTS:

2 sticks salted butter

⅔ cup heavy cream

⅔ cup monk fruit sweetener

½ teaspoon xanthan gum

2 cups pecans, chopped

Sea salt

## DIRECTIONS:

1.  Prepare a cookie sheet with parchment paper or a silicone baking mat.

2.  In a medium-size, medium weight saucepan, brown the butter until it smells nutty. Don't burn the butter. This will take about 5 minutes.

3.  Stir in heavy cream, xanthan gum, and sweetener.

4.  Take the pan off the heat and stir in the nuts.

5.  Place pan in the refrigerator for an hour.

6.  Stir the mixture occasionally while it is getting colder.

7.  After an hour, scoop the mixture onto the cookie sheets and shape into cookies.

8.  Sprinkle with sea salt.

9.  Refrigerate on the cookies sheet until the pralines are hard.

10. After the cookies are hard, transfer to an airtight container in the refrigerator.

11. This is a special treat. A low carb praline with the fat from the butter and cream is a nice dessert to have on a special occasion that you can work into your day without totally messing up your macros. The monk fruit sweetener is a 1:1 measure, so the texture is not altered by not using sugar. Give them a try, and you will not be disappointed.

## NUTRITION:

Calories: 338; Fat: 36g; Protein: 2g; Carbohydrates: 1g.

# RASPBERRY PUDDING SURPRISE

PREPARATION TIME: 20 MINUTES  |  COOKING TIME: 20 MINUTES  |  SERVINGS: 1 SERVING

**INGREDIENTS:**

3 tablespoons chia seeds

½ cup unsweetened almond milk

1 scoop chocolate protein powder

¼ cup raspberries, fresh or frozen

1 teaspoon honey

**DIRECTIONS:**

1. Combine the almond milk, protein powder and chia seeds together.

2. Let rest for 5 minutes before stirring.

3. Refrigerate for 30 minutes.

4. Top with raspberries. Serve!

**NUTRITION:**

Calories: 225; Fat: 21g; Protein: 3g; Carbohydrates: 3g.

# WHITE CHOCOLATE BERRY CHEESECAKE

PREPARATION TIME: 10 MINUTES  |  COOKING TIME: 0 MINUTES  |  SERVINGS: 4 SERVINGS

## INGREDIENTS:

8 ounces cream cheese, softened

2 ounces heavy cream

½ teaspoon Splenda

1 teaspoon raspberries

1 tablespoon Da Vinci Sugar-Free syrup, white chocolate flavor

## DIRECTIONS:

1.  Whip together the ingredients to a thick consistency.

2.  Divide into cups.

3.  Refrigerate.

4.  Serve!

## NUTRITION:

Calories: 330; Fat: 29g; Protein: 6g; Carbohydrates: 6g.

# CONDIMENTS, SAUCES, AND SPREADS RECIPES

## CURRY POWDER

PREPARATION TIME: 10 MINUTES | COOKING TIME: 10 MINUTES | SERVINGS: 20

### INGREDIENTS:

¼ cup coriander seeds

2 tablespoons mustard seeds

2 tablespoons cumin seeds

2 tablespoons anise seeds

1 tablespoon whole allspice berries

1 tablespoon fenugreek seeds

5 tablespoons ground turmeric

### DIRECTIONS:

1. In a large nonstick frying pan, place all the spices except turmeric over medium heat and cook for about 9-10 minutes or until toasted completely, stirring continuously.
2. Remove the frying pan from heat and set aside to cool.
3. In a spice grinder, add the toasted spices and turmeric, and grind until a fine powder forms.
4. Transfer into an airtight jar to preserve.

### NUTRITION:

Calories: 18; Fat: 0.8g; Protein: 0.8g; Carbohydrates: 2.7g.

# POULTRY SEASONING

PREPARATION TIME: 5 MINUTES  |  COOKING TIME: 0 MINUTES  |  SERVINGS: 10

## INGREDIENTS:

2 teaspoons dried sage, crushed finely

1 teaspoon dried marjoram, crushed finely

¾ teaspoon dried rosemary, crushed finely

1 ½ teaspoons dried thyme, crushed finely

½ teaspoon ground nutmeg

½ teaspoon ground black pepper

## DIRECTIONS:

1. Add all the ingredients to a bowl and stir to combine.

2. Transfer into an airtight jar to preserve.

## NUTRITION:

Calories: 2; Fat: 0.1g; Protein: 0.1g; Carbohydrates: 0.4g.

# BASIL PESTO

PREPARATION TIME: 10 MINUTES  |  COOKING TIME: 0 MINUTES  |  SERVINGS: 6

## INGREDIENTS:

2 cups fresh basil

4 garlic cloves, peeled

2/3 cup Parmesan cheese, grated

1/3 cup pine nuts

½ cup olive oil

Salt and ground black pepper, as required

## DIRECTIONS:

1.  Place the basil, garlic, Parmesan cheese, and pine nuts in a food processor, and pulse until a chunky mixture is formed.

2.  While the motor is running gradually, add the oil and pulse until smooth.

3.  Now, add the salt and black pepper, and pulse until well combined.

4.  Serve immediately.

## NUTRITION:

Calories: 232; Fat: 24.2g; Protein: 5g; Carbohydrates: 1.9g.

# BBQ SAUCE

PREPARATION TIME: 15 MINUTES  |  COOKING TIME: 20 MINUTES  |  SERVINGS: 20

## INGREDIENTS:

2 ½ (6-ounce) cans sugar-free tomato paste

½ cup organic apple cider vinegar

1/3 cup powdered erythritol

2 tablespoons Worcestershire sauce

1 tablespoon liquid smoke

2 teaspoons smoked paprika

1 teaspoon garlic powder

½ teaspoon onion powder

Salt, as required

¼ teaspoon red chili powder

¼ teaspoon cayenne pepper

1 ½ cups water

## DIRECTIONS:

1.  Add all the ingredients (except the water) to a pan and beat until well combined.
2.  Add 1 cup of water and beat until combined.
3.  Add the remaining water and beat until well combined.
4.  Place the pan over medium-high heat and bring to a gentle boil.
5.  Adjust the heat to medium-low and simmer, uncovered for about 20 minutes, stirring frequently.
6.  Remove the pan of sauce from the heat and set aside to cool slightly before serving.
7.  You can preserve this sauce in the refrigerator by placing it into an airtight container.

## NUTRITION:

Calories: 22; Fat: 0.1g; Protein: 1g; Carbohydrates: 4.7g.

# KETCHUP

PREPARATION TIME: 10 MINUTES  |  COOKING TIME: 30 MINUTES  |  SERVINGS: 12

## INGREDIENTS:

6 ounces sugar-free tomato paste

1 cup water

¼ cup powdered erythritol

3 tablespoons balsamic vinegar

½ teaspoon garlic powder

½ teaspoon onion powder

¼ teaspoon paprika

1/8 teaspoon ground cloves

1/8 teaspoon mustard powder

Salt, as required

## DIRECTIONS:

1. Add all ingredients to a small pan and beat until smooth.

2. Now, place the pan over medium heat and bring to a gentle simmer, stirring continuously.

3. Adjust the heat to low and simmer, covered for about 30 minutes or until desired thickness, stirring occasionally.

4. Remove the pan from heat and with an immersion blender, blend until smooth.

5. Now, set aside to cool completely before serving.

6. You can preserve this ketchup in the refrigerator by placing it in an airtight container.

## NUTRITION:

Calories: 13; Fat: 0.1g; Protein: 0.7g; Carbohydrates: 2.9g.

# CRANBERRY SAUCE

PREPARATION TIME: 10 MINUTES  |  COOKING TIME: 15 MINUTES  |  SERVINGS: 6

## INGREDIENTS:

12 ounces fresh cranberries

1 cup powdered erythritol

¾ cup water

1 teaspoon fresh lemon zest, grated

½ teaspoon organic vanilla extract

## DIRECTIONS:

1. Place the cranberries, water, erythritol, and lemon zest in a medium pan and mix well.
2. Place the pan over medium heat and bring to a boil.
3. Adjust the heat to low and simmer for about 12-15 minutes, stirring frequently.
4. Remove the pan from heat and mix in the vanilla extract.
5. Set aside at room temperature to cool completely.
6. Transfer the sauce into a bowl and refrigerate to chill before serving.

## NUTRITION:

Calories: 32; Fat: 0.2g; Protein: 0g; Carbohydrates: 5.3g.

# YOGURT TZATZIKI

PREPARATION TIME: 10 MINUTES | COOKING TIME: 0 MINUTES | SERVINGS: 12

**INGREDIENTS:**

1 large English cucumber, peeled and grated

Salt, as required

2 cups plain Greek yogurt

1 tablespoon fresh lemon juice

4 garlic cloves, minced

1 tablespoon fresh mint leaves, chopped

2 tablespoons fresh dill, chopped

Pinch of cayenne pepper

Ground black pepper, as required

**DIRECTIONS:**

1.  Arrange a colander in the sink.

2.  Place the cucumber into the colander and sprinkle with salt.

3.  Let it drain for about 10-15 minutes.

4.  With your hands, squeeze the cucumber well.

5.  Place the cucumber and remaining ingredients in a large bowl and stir to combine.

6.  Cover the bowl and place in the refrigerator to chill for at least 4-8 hours before serving.

**NUTRITION:**

Calories: 36; Fat: 0.6g; Protein: 2.7g; Carbohydrates: 4.5g.

# ALMOND BUTTER

PREPARATION TIME: 10 MINUTES   |   COOKING TIME: 15 MINUTES   |   SERVINGS: 8

## INGREDIENTS:

2 ¼ cups raw almonds

1 tablespoon coconut oil

¾ teaspoon salt

4-6 drops liquid stevia

½ teaspoon ground cinnamon

## DIRECTIONS:

1. Preheat your oven to 325°F.

2. Arrange the almonds onto a rimmed baking sheet in an even layer.

3. Bake for about 12-15 minutes.

4. Remove the almonds from the oven and let them cool completely.

5. In a food processor, fitted with a metal blade, place the almonds and pulse until a fine meal forms.

6. Add the coconut oil and salt, and pulse for about 6-9 minutes.

7. Add the stevia and cinnamon, and pulse for about 1-2 minutes.

8. You can preserve this almond butter in the refrigerator by placing it into an airtight container.

## NUTRITION:

Calories: 170; Fat: 15.1; Protein: 5.7g; Carbohydrates: 5.8g.

# LEMON CURD SPREAD

PREPARATION TIME: 10 MINUTES | COOKING TIME: 10 MINUTES | SERVINGS: 20

## INGREDIENTS:

3 large organic eggs

½ cup powdered erythritol

¼ cup fresh lemon juice

2 teaspoons lemon zest, grated

4 tablespoons butter, cut into 3 pieces

## DIRECTIONS:

1. In a glass bowl, place the eggs, erythritol, lemon juice, and lemon zest.
2. Arrange the glass bowl over a pan of barely simmering water and soak for about 10 minutes or until the mixture becomes thick, beating continuously.
3. Remove from heat and immediately stir in the butter.
4. Set aside for about 2-3 minutes.
5. With a wire whisk, beat until smooth and creamy.

## NUTRITION:

Calories: 32; Fat: 3.1; Protein: 1g; Carbohydrates: 0.2g.

# TAHINI SPREAD

PREPARATION TIME: 10 MINUTES | COOKING TIME: 0 MINUTES | SERVINGS: 4

## INGREDIENTS:

¼ cup tahini

2 garlic cloves, peeled

3 tablespoons olive oil

3 tablespoons water

1 ½ tablespoons fresh lemon juice

¼ teaspoon ground cumin

Salt and ground black pepper, as required

## DIRECTIONS:

1. Place all of the ingredients in a high-speed blender and pulse until creamy.
2. Pour the smoothie into two glasses and serve immediately.

## NUTRITION:

Calories: 183; Fat: 18.7; Protein: 2.7g; Carbohydrates: 3.9g.

# MEASUREMENT AND CONVERSIONS

| CUPS | OZ | G | TBSP | TSP | ML |
|------|------|-----|------|-----|-----|
| 1 | 8 | 225 | 16 | 48 | 250 |
| 3/4 | 6 | 170 | 12 | 36 | 175 |
| 2/3 | 5 | 140 | 11 | 32 | 150 |
| 1/2 | 4 | 115 | 8 | 24 | 125 |
| 1/3 | 3 | 70 | 5 | 16 | 70 |
| 1/4 | 2 | 60 | 4 | 12 | 60 |
| 1/8 | 1 | 30 | 2 | 6 | 30 |
| 1/16 | 1/2 | 15 | 1 | 3 | 15 |

| 250°F | 300°F | 325°F | 350°F | 400°F | 450°F |
|-------|-------|-------|-------|-------|-------|
| 120°C | 150°F | 160°C | 175°C | 200°C | 230°C |

Made in the USA
Middletown, DE
28 November 2021

53667974R00068